The Palgrave Macmillan Animal Ethics Series

Series Editors

Andrew Linzey
Oxford Centre for Animal Ethics
Oxford, UK

Clair Linzey
Oxford Centre for Animal Ethics
Oxford, UK

In recent years, there has been a growing interest in the ethics of our treatment of animals. Philosophers have led the way, and now a range of other scholars have followed from historians to social scientists. From being a marginal issue, animals have become an emerging issue in ethics and in multidisciplinary inquiry. This series will explore the challenges that Animal Ethics poses, both conceptually and practically, to traditional understandings of human-animal relations. Specifically, the Series will:

- provide a range of key introductory and advanced texts that map out ethical positions on animals;
- publish pioneering work written by new, as well as accomplished, scholars;
- produce texts from a variety of disciplines that are multidisciplinary in character or have multidisciplinary relevance.

For further information or to submit a proposal for consideration, please contact Amy Invernizzi, amy.invernizzi@palgrave-usa.com.

More information about this series at
https://link.springer.com/bookseries/14421

Nico Dario Müller

Kantianism for Animals

A Radical Kantian Animal Ethic

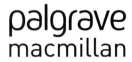

Nico Dario Müller
University of Basel
Basel, Switzerland

ISSN 2634-6672 ISSN 2634-6680 (electronic)
ISBN 978-3-031-01932-6 ISBN 978-3-031-01930-2 (eBook)
https://doi.org/10.1007/978-3-031-01930-2

© The Editor(s) (if applicable) and The Author(s) 2022 This book is an open access publication.

Open Access This book is licensed under the terms of the Creative Commons Attribution 4.0 International License (http://creativecommons.org/licenses/by/4.0/), which permits use, sharing, adaptation, distribution and reproduction in any medium or format, as long as you give appropriate credit to the original author(s) and the source, provide a link to the Creative Commons licence and indicate if changes were made.

The images or other third party material in this book are included in the book's Creative Commons licence, unless indicated otherwise in a credit line to the material. If material is not included in the book's Creative Commons licence and your intended use is not permitted by statutory regulation or exceeds the permitted use, you will need to obtain permission directly from the copyright holder.

The use of general descriptive names, registered names, trademarks, service marks, etc. in this publication does not imply, even in the absence of a specific statement, that such names are exempt from the relevant protective laws and regulations and therefore free for general use.
The publisher, the authors and the editors are safe to assume that the advice and information in this book are believed to be true and accurate at the date of publication. Neither the publisher nor the authors or the editors give a warranty, expressed or implied, with respect to the material contained herein or for any errors or omissions that may have been made. The publisher remains neutral with regard to jurisdictional claims in published maps and institutional affiliations.

Cover illustration: Frank Bienewald / Alamy Stock Photo

This Palgrave Macmillan imprint is published by the registered company Springer Nature Switzerland AG.
The registered company address is: Gewerbestrasse 11, 6330 Cham, Switzerland

NOTE ON REFERENCES, QUOTATIONS, AND TRANSLATIONS

For all references to the works of Immanuel Kant, I use the standard pagination of the *Akademie-Ausgabe*. References consist of an abbreviation of the work's title, followed by the volume of the *Akademie-Ausgabe*, the page number, and usually the line number. For example, "MM 6:442.04-06" refers to the *Metaphysics of Morals*, volume 6 of the *Akademie-Ausgabe*, page 442, lines 4 to 6. An exception is the *Critique of Pure Reason*, for which it is customary to designate the edition (A or B), followed by the page number, but no line numbers (Timmermann 2007, ix). For instance, "CPR B326" refers to the *Critique of Pure Reason*, B-edition, page 326. References to lecture notes of Kant's students use the name of the student, followed by the volume and page number of the *Akademie-Ausgabe*. For example, Collins 27:460 refers to page 460 of Collins's notes, contained in volume 27.

The abbreviations are as follows: *Beobachtungen* = "*Beobachtungen über das Gefühl des Schönen und Erhabenen*", 2:205–256; *Syllogismen* = "*Die falsche Spitzfindigkeit der vier syllogistischen Figuren*", 2:45–61; CPR = "*Kritik der reinen Vernunft*", 3:01–4:252; CPrR = "*Kritik der praktischen Vernunft*", 5:01–163; CPJ = "*Kritik der Urteilskraft*", 5:165–485; Rel = "*Die Religion innerhalb der Grenzen der blossen Vernunft*", 6:01–202; MM = "*Die Metaphysik der Sitten*", 6:203–493; Anth = "*Anthropologie in pragmatischer Hinsicht*", 7:117–333; *Muthmaßlicher Anfang* = "*Muthmaßlicher Anfang der Menschengeschichte*", 8:107–123; *Gemeinspruch* = "*Über den Gemeinspruch: Das mag in der Theorie richtig sein, taugt aber nicht für die Praxis*", 8:273–313;

Jäsche = "*Immanuel Kant's Logik—Ein Handbuch zu Vorlesungen*", 9:001–150; *Nachlaß-Anthropologie* = "*Handschriftlicher Nachlaß: Anthropologie*", 15:V-982.

While references to Kant refer to his original German text, I quote Kant in English throughout. I use the translations published in the *Cambridge Edition* (Gregor 1996; Wood and Di Giovanni 1996; Heath and Schneewind 1997; Guyer 2000; Zöller and Louden 2007), unless indicated otherwise. An exception is Kant's *Tugendlehre*, for which I was kindly given permission to use Gregor, Timmermann, and Grenberg's new translation (Gregor, Timmermann & Grenberg forthcoming). For any English quotations, the page and line numbers still refer to Kant's original German text in the *Akademie-Ausgabe*.

A note on gendered pronouns in translations: A debate exists on whether it is accurate to translate Kant's '*Mensch*' as 'man', and the pronouns that attach to '*Mensch*' as 'he'. After all, '*Mensch*' translates literally to 'human being', without having a connotation of masculinity like the English word 'man' (Kleingeld 2019, 12 f.). The *Cambridge Edition* usually chooses 'human being' instead of 'man' but does use 'he' for the associated pronoun. I do not change the translations in this regard. As Kleingeld points out, there is ample evidence that Kant, objectionably, primarily has men in mind when he talks about '*Menschen*' (Kleingeld 2019, 13). Instead of simply whitewashing the text in the course of translation, Kleingeld suggests we should make Kant's preoccupation with men transparent. This makes for a more honest representation of Kant's views, and it makes it easier to reflect on, and avoid inadvertently replicating, his sexism (Kleingeld 2019, 16–20).

References

Gregor, Mary J., ed. 1996. *Immanuel Kant: Practical philosophy.* Translated by Mary J. Gregor. Cambridge: Cambridge University Press.

Gregor, Mary J., Timmermann, Jens, and Jeanine Grenberg, ed. forthcoming. *Immanuel Kant: The Doctrine of Virtue.* Translated by Mary J. Gregor, Jens Timmermann, and Jeanine Grenberg. Cambridge: Cambridge University Press.

Guyer, Paul, ed. 2000. *Immanuel Kant: Critique of the Power of Judgment.* Translated by Paul Guyer and Eric Matthews. Cambridge: Cambridge University Press.

Heath, Peter, and Jerome B. Schneewind, ed. 1997. *Immanuel Kant: Lectures on ethics.* Translated by Peter Heath. Cambridge: Cambridge University Press.

Kleingeld, Pauline. 2019. On dealing with Kant's sexism and racism. *SGIR Review* 2: 3–22.

Timmermann, Jens. 2007. *Kant's Groundwork of the Metaphysics of Morals: A commentary.* Cambridge: Cambridge University Press.

Wood, Allen W., and George Di Giovanni, ed. 1996. *Immanuel Kant: Religion and rational theology.* Translated by Allen W. Wood and George Di Giovanni. Cambridge: Cambridge University Press.

Zöller, Günter, and Robert B. Louden, ed. 2007. *Immanuel Kant: Anthropology, history, and education.* Translated by Mary J. Gregor, Paul Guyer, Robert B. Louden, Holly L. Wilson, Allen W. Wood, Günter Zöller, and Arnulf Zweig. Cambridge: Cambridge University Press.

Series Editors' Preface

This is a new book series for a new field of inquiry: Animal Ethics.

In recent years, there has been a growing interest in the ethics of our treatment of animals. Philosophers have led the way, and now a range of other scholars have followed from historians to social scientists. From being a marginal issue, animals have become an emerging issue in ethics and in multidisciplinary inquiry.

In addition, a rethink of the status of animals has been fuelled by a range of scientific investigations which have revealed the complexity of animal sentiency, cognition and awareness. The ethical implications of this new knowledge have yet to be properly evaluated, but it is becoming clear that the old view that animals are mere things, tools, machines or commodities cannot be sustained ethically.

But it is not only philosophy and science that are putting animals on the agenda. Increasingly, in Europe and the United States, animals are becoming a political issue as political parties vie for the "green" and "animal" vote. In turn, political scientists are beginning to look again at the history of political thought in relation to animals, and historians are beginning to revisit the political history of animal protection.

As animals grow as an issue of importance, so there have been more collaborative academic ventures leading to conference volumes, special journal issues, indeed new academic animal journals as well. Moreover, we have witnessed the growth of academic courses, as well as university posts, in Animal Ethics, Animal Welfare, Animal Rights, Animal Law, Animals and Philosophy, Human-Animal Studies, Critical Animal Studies, Animals and Society, Animals in Literature, Animals and Religion—tangible signs that a new academic discipline is emerging.

"Animal Ethics" is the new term for the academic exploration of the moral status of the non-human—an exploration that explicitly involves a focus on what we owe animals morally, and which also helps us to understand the influences—social, legal, cultural, religious and political—that legitimate animal abuse. This series explores the challenges that Animal Ethics poses, both conceptually and practically, to traditional understandings of human-animal relations.

The series is needed for three reasons: (1) to provide the texts that will service the new university courses on animals; (2) to support the increasing number of students studying and academics researching in animal related fields, and (3) because there is currently no book series that is a focus for multidisciplinary research in the field.

Specifically, the series will

- provide a range of key introductory and advanced texts that map out ethical positions on animals;
- publish pioneering work written by new, as well as accomplished, scholars, and
- produce texts from a variety of disciplines that are multidisciplinary in character or have multidisciplinary relevance.

The new Palgrave Macmillan Series on Animal Ethics is the result of a unique partnership between Palgrave Macmillan and the Ferrater Mora Oxford Centre for Animal Ethics. The series is an integral part of the mission of the Centre to put animals on the intellectual agenda by facilitating academic research and publication. The series is also a natural complement to one of the Centre's other major projects, the *Journal of Animal Ethics*. The Centre is an independent "think tank" for the advancement of progressive thought about animals, and is the first Centre of its kind in the world. It aims to demonstrate rigorous intellectual enquiry and the highest standards of scholarship. It strives to be a world-class centre of academic excellence in its field.

We invite academics to visit the Centre's website www.oxfordanimaleth-ics.com and to contact us with new book proposals for the series.
Andrew Linzey and Clair Linzey
General Editors

Oxford, UK   Andrew Linzey
Oxford, UK   Clair Linzey

ACKNOWLEDGEMENTS

This book is the result of my dissertation project at the University of Basel, funded by the Swiss National Science Foundation's Doc.CH programme (grant number P0BSP1_172427). The publication was further supported by the SNSF NCCR Evolving Language (agreement number 51NF40_180888) and an SNSF Open Access Grant (grant number 10BP12_208394). I would like to thank the Swiss National Science Foundation for its support of the project and the open access publication, and the Philosophical Seminar of the University of Basel for hosting and supporting me.

My gratitude belongs to my PhD supervisors, Markus Wild (University of Basel) and Jens Timmermann (University of St Andrews), for their trust in the project, as well as their care, advice, and feedback. I would also like to give special thanks to my colleague Lucas Sierra Vélez for our many discussions about Kantian animal ethics. For his encouragement and kind help with the book publication, I would like to thank series editor Andrew Linzey.

For constructive comments on parts of this book and various helpful discussions, I am grateful to Muriel Leuenberger, Friederike Zenker, Bettina Huber, Michael O'Leary, Angela Martin, Lukas Hilgert, Dominique Hosch, Deborah Mühlebach, Matthieu Queloz, Jelscha Schmid, Anne Meylan, Melanie Sarzano, Marie van Loon, Rebekka Hufendiek, Christine Sievers, Hannah Fasnacht, Colin King, Samuel Tscharner, Marc Sommer, Federica Basaglia, Samuel Camenzind, Saskia Stucki, Johannes Nickl, Stefano Lo Re, Jannis Schaab, Pärttyli Rinne,

Michael Walschots, Ben Sachs, Martin Sticker, Leif Wenar, Anita Leirfall, Philipp Hagen, Adrian Häfliger, and Stefan Riedener.

For their support, interest, and patience over the last years, I would like to thank my partner Carol Zahnd, my family Judith Sidler, Franco Müller, Silvia Sidler, Luisa Müller, Lina Müller, Matthias Steinmann, Sara Zahnd, and Andreas Zahnd, as well as my friends and animal advocacy collaborators Pablo Labhardt, Céline Schlegel, Niklaus Schneider, Delia Hasler, Larissa Schmidt, Nicolas Eichenberger, and Matthias Meier. For tripping over him in the middle of the night, I would like to apologise to my black cat Kiki (see Sect. 5.4 below).

PRAISE FOR *KANTIANISM FOR ANIMALS*

"*Kantianism for Animals* is an excellent book. In rigorous yet accessible prose, it clearly explains how Kantian ethics works, what makes this theory compelling, and what makes this theory compatible with a radical vision for animal rights. Kantians and non-Kantians alike will benefit from reading this book and incorporating its many insights into their thinking about what we owe other animals."
—Jeff Sebo, *Affiliated Professor of Bioethics, Medical Ethics, Philosophy, and Law, New York University, USA*

"Müller's arguments merit attention from Kantians generally, not only from those seeking to establish duties to animals. Noteworthy aspects of Müller's approach include his distinction between bases of moral respect and moral concern, his account of the directionality of ethical duties, his grounding duties to animals in the obligatory end of others' happiness, and his exclusively first-personal account of the authority of morality."
—Lara Denis, *Professor of Philosophy, Agnes Scott College, USA*

"This is a very original contribution that does something quite different from previous animal-friendly versions of Kantianism, say as found in books by Tom Regan or Christine Korsgaard. The author has considered all of the recent scholarship as well as Kant's texts themselves. Further, Müller treats in detail nuanced distinctions made by Kant that are frequently either ignored or misunderstood."
—Daniel A. Dombrowski, *Professor of Philosophy, Seattle University, USA*

"With this book, Nico Müller proposes a completely new approach to Kantian animal ethics. His argument has the great advantage of reading the Kantian text competently and rigorously, avoiding instrumental interpretations of Kant's thought. His 'Kantianism for Animals' is one of the most convincing proposals so far advanced for a deontological approach in animal and environmental ethics."
Federica Basaglia, *Lecturer in Philosophy, University of Konstanz, Germany*

"This original work is a major contribution to the field of Kantian animal ethics. Müller's *revisionist* approach challenges popular readings and shows how *constructive* an adjusted version of Kantianism can be for animal ethics. His *radical* agenda is an imperative for Kantians and animal ethicists. Müller argues in a careful and refreshingly original way that animals merit moral attention, in the same way and for the same reasons as human beings."
—Samuel Camenzind, *Senior Scientist, University of Vienna, Austria*

CONTENTS

List of Tables

PART I

Kantian Foundations

CHAPTER 1

What Is Promising About a Radical Kantian Animal Ethic

1.1   KANTIANISM FOR ANIMALS

Under a certain description, Immanuel Kant appears like an intellectual ancestor of today's animal rights movement.[1] Here we have a philosopher who insists that duty trumps self-interest. That we should treat others according to rational principles, not momentary appetites. That moral responsibility arises from the capacity to determine our own actions autonomously—not from tradition, a self-interested contract with other human beings, or the commands of a human-shaped God. That we should exercise self-control. That we should not exalt ourselves above others. That we should cultivate sympathy and act on it. Even—though this is less widely

---

[1] In animal ethics, it is customary to note that one uses 'animals' as a shorthand for 'non-human animals'. But for my purposes, this seems too strict and too loose. It is too strict because the ethical framework proposed in this book treats other human beings and animals largely equally, and so its application is not restricted to *non-human* animals. It is too loose because Kantian moral concern for others, on my reading, is a matter of regard for their *happiness* on a broadly hedonistic conception (see Sect. 2.3 below). So *non-sentient animals* cannot be objects of this kind of concern. Explicitly using 'animal' as a shorthand for 'non-human animal' turns a vague, everyday notion into a more specific, biological notion, and one which unhelpfully lumps together pigs, orang-utans, drosophilae, sponges, and corals. What I have in mind when I say 'animal' is *a being capable of happiness*, where 'happiness' is a function of hedonic states (see Sect. 2.3). I take it that this coincides roughly with the beings we usually think of first when we talk about 'animals', except that it also includes human beings.

© The Author(s) 2022
N. D. Müller, *Kantianism for Animals*, The Palgrave Macmillan
Animal Ethics Series,
https://doi.org/10.1007/978-3-031-01930-2_1

known—that we should adopt the happiness of others, along with our own moral integrity, as the supreme ends of our actions. Do today's ethical vegans and animal advocates not think along these lines? I know I do. Us friends of animals may disagree with the eighteenth-century Prussian professor on what exactly our duties are, but our movement takes a general view of morality that seems to hew close to his. So we might draw great benefit from considering our own moral thinking through the lens of Kant's philosophical framework of notions, distinctions, and arguments. For one thing, better understanding our own moral thinking helps us remain critical and inquisitive. But it is also crucial when trying to convince others.

Alas, the above description of Kant is selective. In other passages, he appears harshly dismissive of animals. Most importantly, he denied that human beings have any duties whatsoever towards animals (MM 6:442.08–12; MM 6:241.10–17; *Collins* 27:460). We do bear a moral responsibility to treat animals with a certain sympathy, since sympathy in general is an important capacity in our moral relations with other human beings (MM 6:443.13–16). But we have this responsibility only towards ourselves, not the animals. Kant explicitly states that his anthropocentric view does not rule out killing animals for food, coercing them into labour, and using them in scientific experiments (if these experiments serve a human purpose over and above mere speculation, MM 6:443.16–21). According to Kant, the human being is "the ultimate end of the creation here on earth" (CPJ 5:426.36–37), animals are merely "things […] with which one can do as one likes" (Anth 127.08–09). For all his 'Copernican Revolutions', Kant never came to view the doctrine of human superiority as a convenient human rationalisation.

In recent years, this aspect of Kant's philosophy has been unpopular. Even sympathetic readers have called Kant's denial of duties to animals "counterintuitive", "repugnant", "notorious", "unsettling", "entirely unsatisfactory", "inadequate", and "offensive".[2] Although, as we will see, there remain influential voices in the debate who defend and laud Kant for his supposed insight that animals do not matter for their own sake, it is dawning on more and more readers that Kant's views on animals stand in dire need of revision.

---

[2] In the order of appearance: "counterintuitive" (Potter 2005, 303), "repugnant" (Hill 1994, 58), "notorious" (Wood 1998, 189), "unsettling" (O'Hagan 2009, 531), "entirely unsatisfactory" (Calhoun 2015, 194), "inadequate and offensive" (Timmermann 2005, 128).

When animal ethicists write about Kant, they rarely say more than that he denied the existence of duties to animals. To many, this implication makes Kant's entire approach to moral philosophy untenable (Broadie and Pybus 1974; Skidmore 2001; Moyer 2001; Regan 2004, 174–185; Wolf 2012). Animal ethicists tend to see Kant the way they see a Descartes or a Malebranche, namely as a relic from a darker philosophical age that we can happily leave to history. But this perspective on Kant fails to appreciate the philosophical commonalities he shares with today's animal advocates, as well as the positive, creative potential his framework could have for animal ethics. We can only speculate what animal ethicists *could* do with Kant if only they engaged with his thought more where it is helpful. How could an opponent of animal exploitation draw on the notion that we must never use others as mere means? What might change about our understanding of vegetarianism if we based it on autonomy and moral integrity, rather than purely on the avoidance of bad consequences? What relation to wild animals and their environment can one justify with a body of philosophy that asks us to love others, yet not encroach upon them too much? There is a potential for challenging, unusual, and exciting animal ethics here. But as things stand, the way ahead is blocked by Kant's own insistence that our duties can never be directed towards animals. One can hardly blame animal ethicists for refusing to engage with a philosopher who devalues animals out of hand.

But could we go the other way? That is: Instead of rejecting and ignoring Kant's system of moral philosophy, could we develop a new *version* of Kantianism that recognises the existence of duties towards animals? This amended version of Kantianism might still, say, derive duties from our own autonomy rather than from an axiology of pleasure and pain. It might still view duties as primary to moral rights or claims, and acknowledge that we have duties to self. And it might still tie the moral worth of actions to their incentives.[3] But it would not restrict moral consideration to human beings.

When we try to imagine this potential ethical framework, the question arises naturally: In what respects could it remain Kantian 'capital K', and on which underlying issues would it have to differ from Kant? A good answer to this question does two things: First, it explains why Kant excluded animals, thus identifying the points on which we would have to

---

[3] According to my account, all of these points do turn out to be features of Kantianism for Animals. For a summary of the Kantian-for-Animals framework, see Chap. 7.

disagree with him in order to recognise duties towards animals. Secondly and more importantly for animal ethicists, it illuminates an alternative framework, one that remains as close to Kant as possible without denying that there are duties to animals. Call this framework 'Kantianism for Animals'.

Although the strongest reason for developing Kantianism for Animals is its positive potential for animal ethics, there also lies a risk in *not* developing it. The objectionable philosophers that social movements do not reclaim can quickly become the figureheads of their adversaries. In fact, Kant has already had a turbulent history of being claimed by both sides of political animal welfare struggles. First, appeals to Kant's staunchly anthropocentric views of animal ethics were instrumental for the nineteenth-century animal welfare movement in Germany and Great Britain (Altman 2011, 34; Baranzke and Ingensiep 2019, 35). At a time when the very idea of using the law to protect animals was considered novel and unfamiliar, Kant's human-centred considerations against cruelty served as a catalyst. If animal protection was not ultimately about protecting animals, but about protecting human beings, then it might be legitimate to legislate about it. Interestingly enough, it was always Kant's *Doctrine of Virtue* to which animal-friendly politicians and advocates turned, despite the fact that its topic are explicitly non-legal, *ethical* duties (MM 6:388.32–33). So the kind of Kantian argument that most strongly influenced early animal welfare politics did not provide a direct *legal-philosophical* or *political* argument. Its role was rather to lend *ethical* legitimacy to anti-cruelty policies—to tell us why a certain type of treatment of animals is ethically desirable.

More than a century later, the dialectical context has changed dramatically. Under animal welfare regimes inspired by Kant's anthropocentric anti-cruelty doctrine, animal use has been industrialised and expanded to an extent unimaginable in the eighteenth century. To be certain, many countries now have highly detailed animal welfare regulation which outlaws 'unnecessary' or 'cruel' violence. However, most of the violence actually perpetrated against animals—the confining, the injuring, the mutilating, the separating, the killing—is inflicted with the blessing of regulation, since it is considered 'necessary' to achieve some preconceived human purpose. In important ways, the state is still not interested in animals for their own sake, but rather in preventing cruelty from driving human actions. This shows how little we have truly advanced beyond Kant's anthropocentrism.

It is only thanks to the struggle of an ever-growing animal rights movement that we are seeing a slow process of incremental 'subjectivisation' of animal welfare legislation in certain countries (Stucki 2016, 138). That is to say, although these legislations started out protecting animals purely as legal objects, out of human-centred concerns, over time they have granted to animals certain protections for their own sake, a sliver of legal subjecthood. For example, the Swiss constitution and animal welfare law acknowledge that animals have a value in themselves, even calling this value by the Kantian-sounding name "dignity" (Bolliger 2016). Although legislation at this high level is only as good as its concretisation, steps away from pure anthropocentrism are basically a good thing for animals. A law that aims at protecting animal lives and welfare, even if it succeeds only to some extent, can go much further in its prescriptions and prohibitions than a law that aims merely at curtailing human cruelty. For this reason, many animal ethicists today call for the further subjectivisation of legal animal protection, often expressed in terms of animal rights (these are the people I mean when I speak of 'progressive' animal ethicists in this book). The future of the animal rights movement lies in reforming laws and societies for the benefit of the animals themselves, not just for the prevention of cruel character dispositions in human beings.

For the animal rights movement today, Kant's anthropocentrism is a philosophical obstacle and threat. It is an *obstacle* insofar as it legitimises the dominant paradigm of anti-cruelty and animal welfare legislation, which condones and perpetuates the suffering and death of billions of animals each year worldwide, by appeal to a philosophical system that continues to be taken very seriously. It poses a *threat* in that it can easily be weaponised for reactionary anti-animal politics that would rather undo what little progress the animal rights movement has made and give human beings even more licence to exploit animals (so long as they do not recognisably do it with cruel pleasure, of course). It is no coincidence that some of the literature's most ardent opponents of animal rights have made frequent appeals to Kant (Cohen 1997, 2001; Scruton 2006). Since Kant is so closely associated with the notions of reason, freedom, and autonomy, these reactionary appeals also simultaneously serve to stereotype animal advocates as irrational, illiberal, and sentimental.

In the midst of this dialectic, animal advocates concede too much if they reject Kant wholesale. A certain amount of reclaiming is advisable, and other social movements have set good examples for how this can be done. Critical race theorists were the first to point out and investigate

Kant's now-notorious racism against anyone who is not a white northern European (Eze 1995, 1997; Mills 1998; Bernasconi 2002, 2003). But instead of ignoring Kant and leaving him to be appropriated by today's racists, Mills (1998, 2018) has carefully dissected Kant's philosophy and rebuilt it into a "Black Radical Kantianism" (Mills 2018). Similarly, Hay (2013) has shown how Kant, the famous sexist, can still be of use to feminist philosophy—on a certain reading, with certain modifications. On Hay's account, Kant's notion of a duty to self can help us capture the moral predicament of oppressed human beings. We may owe it not only to *others* to resist oppression, but also to *ourselves*. The aim behind such revisions, reclamations, and repurposings of Kant is not to preserve his reputation as a canonical European philosopher. Nor is it a matter of uncritically invoking Kant in order to then adorn social movements with his plumes. To the contrary, a *partial* revision and reclamation of Kant requires a critical engagement with his work. The aim behind such reclamations is to draw on a corpus of philosophical thought—which, for better or worse, is common philosophical currency—to advance the thought of a social movement, in the sense both of refining it and of spreading it. Kant here appears less like a philosophical authority to be revered, but more like a philosophical resource to be put to good use.

We are yet to see the same level of critical and creative engagement with Kant when it comes to his views on animals. When Kant scholars have commented on these views, they have mostly been preoccupied with showing two things: first, that Kant has good theory-internal reasons for his most notorious claims—say, that animals have no intrinsic value (Hay 2020), that animals do not have the same kind of moral standing as human beings (Hayward 1994; Denis 2000; Garthoff 2020), and that we do not have any duties 'towards' animals (Baranzke 2005; Herman 2018; Howe 2019; Ripstein and Tenenbaum 2020; Varden 2020). Secondly, and in the same texts, they argue that the upshots of such views are nevertheless quite animal-friendly. The problem is that they typically make the first point with much more force and precision than the second. Kant scholars are adept at explaining the internal intricacies of Kant's thought, but they are not particularly trained to assess animal ethical implications thoroughly and critically. Nor is it their job to reflect on and endorse any specific agenda in animal politics against which they could measure the appropriateness of Kant's views. Should it turn out, on a closer look, that objectionably animal-*unfriendly* upshots follow from Kant's views, all that is left is a defence of objectionable views in animal ethics. And indeed, I will argue in Chap. 3 that Kant's denial of duties to animals does have troubling implications no matter how charitable we are.

Against this backdrop, this book pursues three goals: first, to investigate what leads Kant to the conclusion that we have no duties towards animals; secondly, to propose a way to include animals in Kantian moral concern, *pace* Kant; and third, to explore where the changes lead us. My claim is that we must disagree with Kant on certain issues if we want to include animals in his conception of moral concern for their own sake, but these disagreements are surprisingly peripheral to his ethical system. In large parts, Kant's moral philosophy survives the conversion to an ethic that recognises duties towards animals.

The result is a coherent and interesting philosophical framework, Kantianism for Animals, on which animal ethicists can draw to reflect on our moral relations to animals. It is a 'radical' system in the sense that it includes animals in Kantian moral concern 'at the root', in the same way and on the same grounds as it includes other human beings. It also lends itself as a starting point for a 'radical' critique of practices such as using and eating animals (see Chaps. 8 and 9) that takes as its object not just the contingent consequences of these practices, but the very ends and incentives from which they spring.

1.2   A Constructive, Revisionist, Radical Agenda

To see more clearly what distinguishes this book from other texts on Kantian animal ethics, consider the origins of the debate. Although Kantian ethics and animal ethics have both flourished in anglophone philosophy since the 1960s, they have flourished in largely separate social biomes. Most of the literature's few dozen articles were written either by professional Kantians making a brief foray into animal ethics, or vice versa. Korsgaard (2004, 2012, 2013, 2018) was the first to pay more than occasional attention to both fields. She was also the first to publish a monograph on Kantian animal ethics (Korsgaard 2018), after which recently followed the field's first edited volume (Callanan and Allais 2020). Although all of these contributions have helped to advance the debate a great deal, the book you are reading takes a different approach to the topic. The approach can be summarised in three words: *constructive*, *revisionist*, and *radical*.

First, this book does not pursue a destructive anti-Kantian project, but a constructive Kantian one. The aim is emphatically *not* to prove Kant's

moral philosophy wrong by way of a *modus tollens* argument about its
unacceptable implications in animal ethics. To do just that has been the
goal of a long series of previous contributions by animal ethicists (Broadie
and Pybus 1974; Pybus and Broadie 1978; Hoff 1983; Skidmore 2001;
Moyer 2001; Regan 2004, 174–185). Of course, considering critical perspectives is indispensable when scrutinising Kant's system, and hence I will
discuss them at various points throughout the book, especially in Chap. 3.
But at the end of the day, a destructive approach has little to offer to animal ethicists. Most in this field *already* believe that Kant is not an interesting philosophical interlocutor. What good does it do to reinforce this
belief? Instead, I intend to show that an amended version of Kantianism
can be fruitful and interesting for animal ethicists. Due to this constructive
approach, I also try to tamper with Kant as little as possible, though as
much as necessary.

Secondly, this book's approach is revisionist, rather than purely exegetical or defensive. In other words, I do not primarily try to explain or defend
Kant's account of animal ethics in the face of objections. My aim is to
revise and repurpose it. A lot has already been written to defend Kant's
anti-cruelty doctrine, typically by Kantians reacting to what they see as ill-
informed criticism from animal ethicists (Hayward 1994; Denis 2000;
Baranzke 2005; Altman 2011, 2019; Svoboda 2012, 2014; Geismann
2016; Wilson 2017; Herman 2018; Howe 2019). Of course, such defences
are relevant to consider if the goal is a fair assessment of Kant. But even the
strongest refutation of objections can only make Kant's views *less repugnant*, not *more useful* or *interesting* to animal ethicists. To make the most
of Kant in animal ethics, we should try to include animals in Kantian moral
concern. Revisionism presupposes both a certain optimism and a certain
pessimism. It presupposes the optimistic view that Kant's ethical system
can be brought to recognise duties towards animals without sacrificing
too much of what makes it attractive in the first place.[4] At the same time,
revisionism implies the pessimistic view that we must *depart* from Kant on

---

[4] Some Kant scholars have objected that supposedly 'Kantian' approaches to animal ethics
have largely abandoned the substance of Kant's views on morality, merely preserving this or
that superficial "keyword" (Geismann 2016, 413FN3; see also Altman 2011, 26; O'Hagan
2009, 554). However, the approaches they criticise do not represent targeted efforts at constructive revisionism—at staying as close to Kant as possible while recognising duties to animals. They were simply texts in animal ethics that employed Kantian vocabulary. Hence, even
if we agree that some previous 'Kantian' proposals differed very significantly from Kant, this
does not doom all future Kantian proposals to the same fate.

some points to yield acceptably animal-friendly conclusions. So this project also differs from earlier contributions that make the case that duties to animals *already* follow from Kant's views, if only we understand them correctly (Wood 1998; Korsgaard 2004, 2012, 2013; Kaldewaij 2013).[5] For reasons I will explain in Chaps. 3, 4, 5, and 6, I am more pessimistic.

Third, this book takes a 'radical' approach to the inclusion of animals in Kantian moral concern. That is, the aim is to revise Kant's account of moral consideration 'at the root' so that it applies to animals, rather than merely adding duties towards animals after the fact. This approach yields an ethical system in which our duties to animals do not belong to a special, separate class, but are simply instances of our duties to others, just like our duties to other human beings. This radical agenda is stronger than mere non-anthropocentrism. Not only do animals merit moral attention for their own sake, but they merit it for their own sake *in the same way and for the same reasons as other human beings*. In Midgley's words: "If you think cruelty wrong in general—which Kant certainly did—it seems devious to say that cruelty to animals is wrong for entirely different reasons from cruelty to people" (Midgley 1995, 33). At the same time, the agenda does not imply that our duties towards human beings and animals are exactly identical in their *demands*, only that they have the same form and normative ground. We can concede that beneficence demands markedly different actions vis à vis bats and human beings, just like beneficence can demand different actions vis à vis human beings with different tastes. But the duty of beneficence is still one and the same towards both.[6]

<hr />

[5] Altman (2011, 26, 35) suggests that Korsgaard and Wood set out to "revise" Kant's views. This strikes me as only half true. Though both Korsgaard and Wood aim to show that Kant was wrong about whether animals are ends in themselves, they each argue on the basis of (what they take to be) Kant's own, unaltered views. More accurate seems the formulation chosen by Basaglia (2018, 90), who characterises Wood and Korsgaard as 'correcting' Kant based on theory-internal Kantian considerations. My own disagreements with Kant, in any case, will not be intended as 'corrections' on his own terms, but as disagreements based on my preconceived, radical approach.

[6] Note that this type of 'radicalism' is still compatible with various views about whether duties to animals and duties to rational human beings are equal in weight. If one considers it a desideratum to give less weight to the claims of animals than those of rational human beings (as Garthoff does, Garthoff 2011, 25), one can still try to account for this imbalance after the fact, particularly within an account on how to resolve apparent moral conflicts. Like Kant's own view, however, Kantianism for Animals will not come with a highly specific view on the resolution of apparent moral conflict (see Chap. 11).

While Kantians have made non-anthropocentric proposals, they have not been radical in this sense. Their main concern was to present a Kantian argument in favour of protecting animals for their own sake, but they are happy to let this argument run along a very different path from its human-centred counterpart.[7] An example is Cholbi's argument that animal welfare is an 'end in itself' because it does not depend on a good will for its goodness (Cholbi 2014, 348). Whereas human happiness is only good if we deserve it, animal welfare is always good (so that a disinterested rational spectator would approve of it). From this value of animal welfare, Cholbi then directly derives duties towards animals (Cholbi 2014, 349). In doing so, his aim is explicitly *not* to set moral concern for human beings and animals on equal footing (Cholbi 2014, 338). After all, Kant's account of our duties towards other human beings does not hinge on any premiss to the effect that their happiness is good independently of a good will, nor does Cholbi think it does. Hence, his view is purposely non-radical (though I will draw on it for my radical purposes, see Chaps. 4 and 6).

Another example of a non-anthropocentric, but non-radical approach is Korsgaard's.[8] As she emphasises herself, "our moral relations to the other animals have a different basis and a different shape than our moral relations to other people" (Korsgaard 2018, 148). The difference is that our duties to other human beings respond to interpersonal moral 'constraint' under a shared moral law, but our duties to animals do not (Korsgaard 2004, 104, 2018, 123–126). Thus, animals 'obligate' us only in a different sense than human beings (Korsgaard 2018, 147), and they are 'ends in themselves' only in a different sense too (Korsgaard 2018, 141). Drawing such distinctions is almost inevitable if duties to animals are put on a different philosophical basis from duties to other human beings. But it can also lead into trouble: If interpersonal constraint accounts for the 'directionality' of our duties—their character of being 'directed towards' others—it appears unclear how our duties towards animals can be directed 'towards' them. They may be duties *about* animals, or duties at which we arrive by considering animal well-being. But in Kant's terminology, these would simply be duties *regarding* animals, not *towards*. Since Korsgaard

---

[7] Other examples of such approaches include Wood (1998), O'Neill (1998), and Garthoff (2011).

[8] Another difference between this book and Korsgaard's is that hers builds upon her own original, neo-Kantian thought. Kant is an inspiration here, to be sure. But a diagnosis of why Kant himself excluded animals and an amendment of his system is simply not Korsgaard's project.

does not reject the notion that directionality requires a shared moral law (Korsgaard 2018, 124), it is hard to see how her 'obligations to the other animals' could be anything else than Kantian 'indirect' duties repackaged.[9] Ultimately, every non-radical account of duties towards animals runs the risk of collapsing back into old-fashioned Kantian anthropocentrism, since the duties we add to Kant's system after the fact fail to be directed towards the animals in the way Kant's duties are directed towards human beings.[10]

Setting such philosophical troubles aside, a radical approach has the added benefit of making Kant's own discussion of our duties more directly relevant to our duties towards animals. If our duties towards animals are not a special and separate class of duty, but the same in form and ground as our duties to human beings, we can repurpose more of Kant's own philosophical tools for animal ethics. So, without denigrating the philosophical and political value of non-radical approaches, there is great potential in pursuing a radical approach.

Apart from its different approach to the topic, there is another feature which sets the present text apart from the previous literature on Kantian animal ethics: Being one of the first *monographs* on the topic to date, it has more space at its disposal, particularly to explore implications concerning some specific questions of animal ethics. We need not content ourselves with showing *that* there can be Kantian duties towards animals, but we can also explore to some extent *what* duties they might be, and what kinds of arguments animal ethicists might construct from considerations about

---

[9] Even if Korsgaard's duties 'towards' animals are ultimately Kantian duties 'regarding' animals, it must be said that in substance, her duties go far beyond Kant's. Still, we have yet to see a version of a Kantian ethic that includes duties to animals in the same way as it includes duties towards other human beings. The driving motivator behind the book you are reading is the desire to explore what such an ethic could look like and what philosophical considerations it could encourage.

[10] The collapse is particularly explicit in Herman (2018). The chapter starts with the mission statement of "figuring out how animals might be brought inside Kantian morality" (Herman 2018, 174). Since Herman subscribes to the view that human moral status is explained by their moral agency (Herman 2018, 178), an *additional* argument is needed to 'make room' for animals in Kant's system of ethics. A mere six pages after stating her mission, Herman arrives at the conclusion: "In lacking the capacity for moral agency, animals cannot be wronged in the way that is marked by violations of duty. In my terms, that makes them not participants in the moral habitat project" (Herman 2018, 180). She proceeds to defend Kant's 'indirect duty' view. In Chap. 3, I will argue that such defences are overstated. In Chap. 4, I will cast doubt on Kantian arguments that attempt to derive human moral patienthood from the conditions of moral agency.

them. Hence, the format of a book makes it easier to illustrate what kind of novel insight can be gained by considering a Kantian perspective—adequately amended—on our moral relations to animals.

1.3   Limitations and Responses to Initial Worries

Even in a book, there is not enough space to discuss all issues at the intersection of Kantian ethics and animal ethics. Some limitations are inevitable, and I want to mention two in particular: First, this book is strictly concerned with the *treatment* of animals, with their role as moral patients rather than moral agents or subjects. This is important not only because animal ethicists take an increasing interest in animals as more active participants in morality (e.g. De Waal 2003, 2006; Bekoff 2004; Bekoff and Pierce 2009; Rowlands 2012). It is also important because it starkly distinguishes this book's project from aforementioned projects in Kantian feminist and anti-racist theory. Both Hay and Mills draw heavily on Kant's views on human beings as moral *agents*. Their liberatory projects rely on strengthening the egalitarian parts of Kant's thinking while revising its racist and sexist structures and commitments. But the move of reemphasising Kant's egalitarianism among autonomous beings will evidently not help animals. They are not 'autonomous' in the sense that matters for Kantian ethics: being able to act on a self-imposed moral law.[11] The problem is thus not that Kant made a mistake in thinking that animals do not meet his system's criteria for moral concern. The problem lies in the criteria themselves. We cannot plausibly include animals in a picture of reciprocal moral relations between autonomous, free, and equal agents. Rather, we need to challenge the very idea that such reciprocity is a necessary feature of Kantian moral relations.[12] To be sure, this limitation is not a bad

[11] Some in the literature rightly point out that animals have 'preference autonomy' (Rocha 2015; Thomas 2016; Judd and Rocha 2017). Martin Balluch has additionally suggested that the capacity for rule-based behaviour makes animals Kantian ends in themselves (Balluch 2016). But none of these capacities are what Kant has in mind when he talks about 'autonomy', which is rather the capacity to act on a self-imposed moral law (see Timmermann 2005, 132).

[12] Note that what is at issue here is the idea that symmetry, reciprocity, or mutuality are *necessary* features of interpersonal moral relations. This is distinct from the idea that such features are *typical* or *characteristic* features of interpersonal moral relations wherever typical, adult human beings are concerned. So whoever finds something attractive in Kant's moral egalitarianism, restricted as it may be, can remain on board with the inclusion of animals.

thing. Rather, the fact that different Kantian considerations are possible with regard to the oppression of autonomous human beings and the oppression of animals might itself tell us something worthwhile about the differences between these types of oppression.

The second limitation is that this book covers only one out of two types of Kantian moral duty. What this book is concerned with are so-called *ethical* duties, which Kant also calls *duties of virtue*. I am not concerned with *legal* duties, which Kant calls *duties of right*. This fundamental distinction is a recurrent theme throughout Kant's later moral philosophy (for more on the distinction see Chap. 2). In short, ethical duties are a matter of 'inner' legislation (MM 6:220.19–21). They prescribe adopting certain ends or maxims, telling us what to *will* or *strive for* rather than what to *do* in terms of purely outward acts. Legal duties, by contrast, are a matter of 'outer' legislation (MM 6:229.05–6). They prescribe mere acts irrespective of motive. Due to this difference, we can *force* others to observe legal duties, but not ethical duties, since we can only force others to perform certain acts, but not to perform them for the sake of some particular end (MM 6:381.30–33; MM 6:383.18–20). Because they are enforceable, legal duties call for a *Doctrine of Right*: an account not only of what we *may do*, but also of what the state or other human beings *may force us* to do. Kant develops this account in the first book of the *Metaphysics of Morals*. But how exactly this *Doctrine of Right* relates to the rest of his moral philosophy is a difficult and controversial question. On one influential reading, legal duties do not derive from the Categorical Imperative at all, but from an entirely separate social contract theory, and hence they do not truly belong in the *Metaphysics of Morals* (Willaschek 1997, 2009). But of course, I do not want to show merely that animals fit into some detachable part of Kant's moral system. Nor is it my goal to argue, against parts of the literature, that legal duties do derive from the Categorical Imperative. This would lead into special exegetical difficulties that have little to do with animals. Therefore, somewhat grudgingly, I exclude legal duties from my view in this book. When I speak of 'moral concern', I always mean the consideration of individuals insofar as there are *ethical* duties towards them (for a justification of this terminology see Chap. 2).

The distinction between ethical and legal duties is perhaps the first piece of helpful Kantian terminology this book can add to the animal ethicist's philosophical toolbox. In later chapters (Chaps. 8, 9, and 10), I hope to show that various interesting arguments can be construed with a Kantian notion of ethical duty particularly because it addresses what we *should will* and not just what we *may do*. The downside of focusing on ethical duties is however that this book cannot offer a *legal-philosophical* or *political* argument for animal rights, or indeed for legal protections of any kind. It cannot show that any particular arrangement of institutions and laws is just and legitimate. This is somewhat unfortunate, since it is one of Kant's shortcomings in animal ethics that he considered the morality of our treatment of animals to be a wholly private affair. The problem is not that Kant did not call for animal protection by law, an idea which only began to take serious hold abroad, in Great Britain, around the time of his death. The problem is that even in retrospect, nothing in Kant's *Doctrine of Right* readily lends itself as a basis for the protection of non-autonomous beings.[13] It is hard to see how a system of legal thought based on respect for the external freedom of autonomous beings (see MM 6:230.29–31) could protect animals, let alone at the expense of human utility. Developing a more compelling Kantian perspective on legal animal protection would therefore be a worthwhile endeavour. Korsgaard (2012, 2013) has started the conversation with her Kantian account of animal rights. But this book is unfortunately not the place to continue it.

However, even if Kantianism for Animals is an approach focused on ethical duties, it is indirectly relevant to animal politics. To reiterate: Kant's own anthropocentric arguments were also neither legal-philosophical nor political, yet they contributed a great deal to legitimising early animal welfare policy *ethically*. Kantianism for Animals responds in kind. The framework may not tell us how we *may* treat animals as a matter of legal and political legitimacy. But it tells us something about the ends a good person should pursue and the kind of coexistence with animals they should strive to develop. In this way, the framework can lend *ethical* legitimacy to a political programme.

The book's endeavour may raise some concerns right from the start. First, one might worry that there is not *one* Kant in whose conception of

---

[13] The best theory-internal option, it seems to me, is to argue for animal protection on 'indirect' grounds, say, by appealing to social stability. I thank Jens Timmermann for this suggestion. My worry is that according to such arguments, animal protection is merely one tool in the toolbox to prevent social disarray, and it should probably be a means of last resort, given that it infringes quite heavily on the external freedom of human beings. Hence, indirect arguments do not seem very promising as a basis for legal animal protection Kantian-style. My preferred approach, which I cannot pursue in this project, would be to argue that the *Doctrine of Right* is detachable from Kant's system and that it can be replaced by a more animal-friendly conception, say, by an interest-based theory of rights.

moral concern we can include animals. There are more than 200 years of reception history associated with Kant's moral philosophy, as well as ongoing exegetical debates. In general, there is little consensus on how to read Kant. However, this book's project does not require that we find the 'one true reading' of Kant's text that settles all exegetical debates. All we need is a reading that facilitates a productive engagement on the part of animal ethicists. So if given the choice, we should go for a less orthodox reading that is more productive, not vice versa (so long as it still passes for a reading *of Kant's text*). If anything, the variety of readings makes it easier to find a version of Kant that is helpful.

One might also take issue with the fact that this book about Kant openly presupposes an agenda: It takes as its starting point the view that there are duties to animals, and that these duties have the same form and ground as duties to other human beings. It then asks how Kant's philosophy can be modified to accommodate these presuppositions. One might expect that such an agenda-driven project is unlikely to treat Kant charitably. However, while it is true that this book combines an exegetical perspective with a critical-argumentative one, the *constructive* aim of the project gives rise to a strong interest to read Kant as charitably as possible. The intended result is an amended Kantian system with which animal ethicists will be interested to engage. And the more compelling Kant turns out to be, the more interesting he is to work with later. Indeed, the revisions of Kant's system I will make are not so much *corrections of philosophical errors* on Kant's part. They rather undo certain *philosophical decisions* made by Kant with which one could reasonably disagree and still remain a Kantian in important respects. As far as this book is concerned, the reason why we should disagree with Kant on underlying issues is *not* that Kant's view is obviously indefensible. The reason is simply that these positions lead to the exclusion of animals, which in turn makes Kant unattractive for animal ethicists to work with. So the combination of openly adhering to an agenda in animal ethics, but wanting to make use of Kant, enables a particularly productive and charitable engagement.

1.4   The Way Ahead

The chapters that follow are grouped into three parts: (I) Kantian Foundations, (II) Building Kantianism for Animals, and (III) Using the Framework. My goal in the first part is to further clarify and motivate the project. In Chap. 2, I begin by presenting Kant's account of moral concern. Kant offers a taxonomy of duties with several crucial distinctions, as well as a series of spotlights on duties he deems particularly important. By considering this taxonomy, it becomes clearer what it means to include animals in Kantian moral concern, and we can get another glimpse of what progressive animal ethicists might gain from a Kantian perspective.

In Chap. 3, I add some critical thoughts on Kant's 'indirect duty' view. I do this because Kantian defences have painted the picture that animal ethicists should find nothing objectionable in Kant's views, correctly understood. This is overly optimistic. Though some traditional objections to Kant's view have been overstated, the same must be said about the Kantian defences. There are serious problems with Kant's 'indirect duty' account.

In Part II of the project, I turn to the question what we must change about Kant's ethical system to turn it into Kantianism for Animals. The first step is to make it clear how Kant establishes the account of moral concern introduced in Chap. 2. How is the line of moral concern to be drawn in Kant's view? That is, where do our duties towards others come from, and towards whom can these duties be directed? The first part of my answer (Chap. 4) will be negative: Contrary to popular readings, specific duties towards others do *not* follow directly from formulas of the Categorical Imperative. The attempt to derive moral concern for others directly from the Formula of Humanity in particular leads into philosophical trouble. I point out that in the *Doctrine of Virtue*, Kant himself derives specific ethical duties by means of a 'doctrine of obligatory ends'. According to this doctrine, our chief duty towards others is to promote their happiness. Our chief duty to self is to promote what Kant calls our own moral perfection. As surprising as it may be, the crucial Kantian question when it comes to animals is *not* whether they are 'ends in themselves'. Rather, it is whether they belong among those whose happiness we should strive to promote.

I discuss Kant's stated reason for excluding animals in Chap. 6. In general, it is true that we ought to promote the happiness of others. But Kant also holds that we can only have duties towards those whose will can 'constrain' us. I endorse the reading that Kant ties interpersonal moral relations to the sharing of the moral law. To say that a duty is directed 'towards' an individual is to say that this individual's sharing of the moral law is necessary to make the duty binding. This account excludes all animals who are not autonomous in the strong sense of sharing the moral law. Here is the first point on which we must truly disagree with Kant if we want to include animals in moral concern. I argue that another, more thoroughly 'first-personal' account of interpersonal moral relations is possible. On the alternative view I propose, a duty *towards* an individual is a duty whose content is *about* that individual in a special way. Duties towards others are *duties to promote their happiness*. Duties towards self are *duties to promote one's own moral perfection*. Once we accept this conception *pace* Kant, duties towards animals are possible again.

As I discuss in Chap. 6, some problems remain: Much of what is characteristic about Kant's account of moral concern—most importantly, the idea of a reconciliation between 'love' and 'respect' for others—can only apply to *subjects of pure practical reason*. First, Kant's 'duties of respect' revolve around the recognition of equality in moral potential (which involves respect for others' humanity). Because other human beings are fundamentally our equals in their potential for good and evil, we should not be arrogant or contemptuous towards them, and neither should we be so overbearingly beneficent towards them that their moral self-esteem suffers from it. None of this appears to apply to animals incapable of morality. My argument, however, is that there is still a duty not to exalt ourselves above animals in certain ways. Not because of any equality in moral potential, but because of the fundamental moral incomparability between moral agents and moral non-agents. A second, quite separate problem is that according to Kant, animals are not *subjects of instrumental practical reason*; indeed they are not agents in any ambitious sense of the word. Because they play no active role in pursuing their own happiness, we cannot react to them in the way Kant asks us to react to human beings. However, I will argue that we can be more generous about animals' practical capacities even within the bounds of Kantian philosophy. If we acknowledge that animals are broadly capable pursuers of their own happiness, we end up with a desirably uniform picture of duties towards human beings and animals. This is the last amendment necessary for Kantianism for Animals.

To conclude Part II, Chap. 7 presents an overview of some features that set Kantianism for Animals apart from other approaches in animal ethics. In particular, I highlight five claims: (1) Our own autonomy is the normative basis of our duties towards animals; (2) Duties have explanatory, epistemic, and normative primacy over rights; (3) We have duties to self as well as towards others; (4) We ought to reconcile practical love for animals with non-exaltation; (5) The moral worth of our actions depends on what end we pursue, on the maxim from which our action springs, and on the incentive on which we act. Taken together, these claims not only differentiate Kantianism for Animals from sentimentalist, utilitarian, virtue-ethical, care-ethical, and contractualist approaches. They also differentiate it from self-avowedly 'deontological' approaches.[14]

Part III delves into possible applications of the resulting framework. My goal is to showcase some of the resources Kantianism for Animals brings to the table in animal ethics. A recurrent theme is that Kantianism for Animals is *radical* in the original sense of the word: It goes to the root of the problem rather than dwelling on contingent consequences. Chapter 8 illustrates this by offering a novel argument against *using* animals based on the revised Kantian framework: When we set out to 'use' animals, we treat some non-moral end of ours as a limiting condition on the promotion of the happiness of animals. This is a stance that is opposed to duty, which Kant calls a 'vice'. This objection to animal use is more fundamental than the usual 'abolitionist' line, which argues for the badness of certain preconditions or consequences of animal use, but not for the badness of animal use itself. Chapter 9 offers a novel argument against *eating* animals. Though our duty not to harm and kill live animals are duties directly towards them, there is also a separate duty towards ourselves not to regard the bodies of the recently deceased as mundane commodities for us to consume. This argument is again more radical than its predecessors in the literature, which focus on the harm that contingently follows from meat consumption. Chapter 10 provides an alternative Kantian approach to environmental protection. *Pace* earlier Kantian contributions, I argue that Kant has a largely exploitative approach to the non-human environment. But once the line of moral concern is moved to include animals, this exploitation is no longer objectionable. Kantianism for Animals calls for a distinctly *zoocentric* environmentalism, which is a

---

[14] I generally avoid the label 'deontology' for the reasons laid out in Timmermann (2015). In animal ethics, as in other fields, the label is typically associated with the view that an action's consequences are irrelevant for its moral worth (e.g. Regan 2004, 144). Kant is then sometimes characterised as espousing an "extreme deontological ethical theory" (ibid.). However, the claim is patently untrue that Kant deems consequences morally *irrelevant*. His primary unit of ethical action-guidance is the *end* we ought to pursue. Ends are the objects we seek to bring about by means of our actions (MM 6:384.33–34)—in other words, intended consequences (or parts thereof). So even though an action's moral *worth* is not determined by its consequences, Kant is very much *interested* in the intended consequences of our actions. In this way, the label 'deontology' favours confusions that I would rather avoid from the outset.

more independent and compelling Kantian interlocutor position for environmental ethicists than earlier Kantian proposals. In particular, the notion of a duty to self helps to deal with some philosophical difficulties of approaches that view the environment exclusively through the lens of the good of sentient beings. Finally, Chap. 11 makes a plea for animal ethicists to take a constructive, revisionist, and radical approach to other philosophers besides Kant. This promotes a historically conscious, but appropriately irreverent, discipline of animal ethics.

REFERENCES

Altman, Matthew C. 2011. *Kant and applied ethics: The ses and limits of Kant's practical philosophy*. Malden, MA: Wiley-Blackwell.

Altman, Matthew C. 2019. Animal suffering and moral salience: A defense of Kant's indirect view. *The Journal of Value Inquiry* 53: 275–288.

Balluch, Martin. 2016. Autonomie bei Hunden: Die Fähigkeit, das eigene Handeln durch selbst gesetzte Zwecke Regeln zu unterwerfen, macht nichtmenschliche Tiere im Kant'schen Sinne zu Zwecken an sich. In *Das Handeln der Tiere: Tierliche Agency im Fokus der Human-Animal Studies*, ed. Sven Wirth, Anett Laue, Markus Kurth, Katharina Dornenzweig, Leonie Bossert, and Karsten Balgar, 203–225. Bielefeld: Transcript.

Baranzke, Heike. 2005. Tierethik, Tiernatur und Moralanthropologie im Kontext von § 17, Tugendlehre. *Kant-Studien* 96: 336–363.

Baranzke, Heike, and Hans W. Ingensiep. 2019. Das Mensch-Tier-Verhältnis in Geschichte, Gesellschaft und Recht: Bestandesaufnahme und neue Perspektiven. In *Haben Tiere Rechte? Aspekte und Dimensionen der Mensch-Tier-Beziehung*, 23–38. Berlin: Bundeszentrale für politische Bildung.

Basaglia, Federica. 2018. Kantische Ansätze. In *Handbuch Tierethik: Grundlagen—Kontexte—Perspektiven*, ed. Johann S. Ach and Dagmar Borchers, 89–94. Stuttgart: J.B. Metzler.

Bekoff, Marc. 2004. Wild justice and fair play: Cooperation, forgiveness, and morality in animals. *Biology and Philosophy* 19: 489–520.

Bekoff, Marc, and Jessica Pierce. 2009. *Wild justice: The moral lives of animals*. Chicago: University of Chicago Press.

Bernasconi, Robert. 2002. Kant as an unfamiliar source of racism. In *Philosophers on race: Critical essays*, ed. Julia K. Ward and Tommy L. Lott, 145–166. Malden, MA: Wiley-Blackwell.

Bernasconi, Robert. 2003. Will the real Kant please stand up. *Radical Philosophy* 117: 13–22.

Bolliger, Gieri. 2016. Legal protection of animal dignity in Switzerland: Status quo and future perspectives. *Animal Law* 22: 311–395.

Broadie, Alexander, and Elizabeth M. Pybus. 1974. Kant's treatment of animals. *Philosophy* 49: 375–383.

Calhoun, Cheshire. 2015. But what about the animals? In *Reason, value and respect: Kantian themes from the philosophy of Thomas E. Hill, Jr.*, ed. Mark Timmons and Robert N. Johnson, 194–214. Oxford: Oxford University Press.

Callanan, John J., and Lucy Allais, ed. 2020. *Kant and animals*. Oxford: Oxford University Press.

Cholbi, Michael. 2014. A direct Kantian duty to animals. *The Southern Journal of Philosophy* 52: 338–358.

Cohen, Carl. 1997. Do animals have rights? *Ethics & Behavior* 7: 91–102.

Cohen, Carl. 2001. In defense of the use of animals. In *The animal rights debate*, ed. Tom Regan, 29–46. Lanham, MD: Rowman & Littlefield.

De Waal, Frans. 2003. Morality and the social instincts: Continuity with the other primates. The Tanner Lectures on Human Values.

De Waal, Frans. 2006. *Primates and philosophers: How morality evolved*. Princeton, NJ: Princeton University Press.

Denis, Lara. 2000. Kant's conception of duties regarding animals: Reconstruction and reconsideration. *History of Philosophy Quarterly* 17: 405–423.

Eze, Emmanuel C. 1995. The color of reason: The idea of "race" in Kant's Anthropology. *The Bucknell Review* 38: 200–241.

Eze, Emmanuel C. 1997. *Race and the enlightenment: A reader*. Malden, MA: Wiley-Blackwell.

Garthoff, Jon. 2011. Meriting concern and meriting respect. *Journal of Ethics & Social Philosophy* 5: 1–28.

Garthoff, Jon. 2020. Against the construction of animal ethical standing. In *Kant and animals*, ed. John J. Callanan and Lucy Allais, 191–212. Oxford: Oxford University Press.

Geismann, Georg. 2016. Kants Moralphilosophie und die Pflichten in Ansehung der Tiere und der vernunftlosen Natur überhaupt. *Jahrbuch für Recht und Ethik* 24: 413–449.

Hay, Carol. 2013. *Kantianism, liberalism, and feminism: Resisting oppression*. New York: Palgrave Macmillan.

Hay, Carol. 2020. What do we owe to animals? Kant on non-intrinsic value. In *Kant and animals*, ed. John J. Callanan and Lucy Allais, 176–190. Oxford: Oxford University Press.

Hayward, Tim. 1994. Kant and the moral considerability of non-rational beings. *Royal Institute of Philosophy Supplement* 36: 129–142.

Herman, Barbara. 2018. We are not alone: A place for animals in Kant's ethics. In *Kant on persons and agency*, ed. Eric Watkins, 174–191. Cambridge: Cambridge University Press.

Hill, Thomas E. 1994. Respect for humanity. The Tanner Lectures on Human Values.

Hoff, Christina. 1983. Kant's invidious humanism. *Environmental Ethics* 5: 63–70.

Howe, Alex. 2019. Why Kant animals have rights? *Journal of Animal Ethics* 9: 137–142.

Judd, David, and James Rocha. 2017. Autonomous pigs. *Ethics and the Environment* 22: 1–18.

Kaldewaij, Frederike. 2013. The animal in morality: Justifying duties to animals in Kantian moral philosophy. Doctoral dissertation, Utrecht University.

Korsgaard, Christine M. 2004. Fellow creatures. The Tanner Lectures on Human Values.

Korsgaard, Christine M. 2012. A Kantian case for animal rights. In *Animal law— Tier und Recht: Developments and perspectives in the 21st century*, ed. Margot Michel, Daniela Kühne, and Julia Hänni, 3–25. Zürich/St. Gallen: DIKE.

Korsgaard, Christine M. 2013. Kantian ethics, animals, and the law. *Oxford Journal of Legal Studies* 33: 629–648.

Korsgaard, Christine M. 2018. *Fellow creatures: Our obligations to the other animals*. Oxford: Oxford University Press.

Midgley, Mary. 1995. *Beast and man: The roots of human nature*. New York: Routledge.

Mills, Charles. 1998. *Blackness visible: Essays on philosophy and race*. Ithaca, NY: Cornell University Press.

Mills, Charles. 2018. Black radical Kantianism. *Res Philosophica* 95: 1–33.

Moyer, Jeanna. 2001. Why Kant and ecofeminism don't mix. *Hypathia* 16: 79–97.

O'Hagan, Emer. 2009. Animals, agency, and obligation in Kantian ethics. *Social Theory and Practice* 35: 531–554.

O'Neill, Onora. 1998. Kant on duties regarding nonrational nature—necessary anthropocentrism and contingent speciesism. *Aristotelian Society Supplementary Volume* 72: 211–228.

Potter, Nelson. 2005. Kant on duties to animals. *Jahrbuch für Recht und Ethik* 13: 299–311.

Pybus, Elizabeth M., and Alexander Broadie. 1978. Kant and the maltreatment of animals. *Philosophy* 53: 560–561.

Regan, Tom. 2004. *The case for animal rights*. Berkeley/Los Angeles: University of California Press.

Ripstein, Arthur, and Sergio Tenenbaum. 2020. Directionality and virtuous ends. In *Kant and animals*, ed. John J. Callanan and Lucy Allais, 139–156. Oxford: Oxford University Press.

Rocha, James. 2015. Kantian respect for minimally rational animals. *Social Theory and Practice* 41: 309–327.

Rowlands, Mark. 2012. *Can animals be moral?* Oxford: Oxford University Press.

Scruton, Roger. 2006. *Animal rights and wrongs*. London: Demos.

Skidmore, James. 2001. Duties to animals: The failure of Kant's moral theory. *The Journal of Value Inquiry* 35: 541–559.

Stucki, Saskia. 2016. *Grundrechte für Tiere: Eine Kritik des geltenden Tierschutzrechts und rechtstheoretische Grundlegung von Tierrechten im Rahmen einer Neupositionierung des Tieres als Rechtssubjekt*. Baden-Baden: Nomos.

Svoboda, Toby. 2012. Duties regarding nature: A Kantian approach to environmental ethics. *Kant Yearbook* 4: 143–163.

Svoboda, Toby. 2014. A reconsideration of indirect duties regarding non-human organisms. *Ethical Theory and Moral Practice* 17: 311–323.

Thomas, Natalie. 2016. *Animal ethics and the autonomous animal self.* New York: Palgrave Macmillan

Timmermann, Jens. 2005. When the tail wags the dog: Animal welfare and indirect duty in Kantian ethics. *Kantian Review* 10: 127–149.

Timmermann, Jens. 2015. What's wrong with "deontology"? *Proceedings of the Aristotelian Society* 115: 75–92.

Varden, Helga. 2020. Kant and moral responsibility to animals. In *Kant and animals,* ed. John J. Callanan and Lucy Allais, 157–175. Oxford: Oxford University Press.

Willaschek, Marcus. 1997. Why the Doctrine of Right does not belong in the Metaphysics of Morals: On some basic distinctions in Kant's moral philosophy. *Jahrbuch für Recht und Ethik* 5: 205–227.

Willaschek, Marcus. 2009. Right and coercion: Can Kant's conception of right be derived from his moral theory? *International Journal of Philosophical Studies* 17: 49–70.

Wilson, Holly L. 2017. The green Kant: Kant's treatment of animals. In *Environmental ethics: Reading in theory and application,* ed. Louis P. Pojman, Paul Pojman, and Katie McShane, 7th ed., 87–95. Belmont, CA: Wadsworth.

Wolf, Ursula. 2012. *Ethik der Mensch-Tier-Beziehung.* Frankfurt am Main: Vittorio Klostermann.

Wood, Allen W. 1998. Kant on duties regarding non-rational nature. *Aristotelian Society Supplementary Volume* 72: 189–210.

CHAPTER 2

Kantian Moral Concern, Love, and Respect

2.1 What Is Moral Concern Kantian-Style?

This book is all about moral concern for animals: How can a Kantian framework account for the view that animals matter morally? To start with, let us consider what it means for *anyone* to 'matter' in Kant's ethics. As stereotypes would have it, Kantian moral concern follows from a sort of moral algorithm. To be an object of moral concern is to fall within the scope of an application of the Categorical Imperative. However, in this chapter I aim to show how Kant's conception of moral concern is at once much richer and much more down-to-earth.[1] This also makes it clearer why Kant's framework could be interesting for animal ethicists to work with.

Kant himself did not use the now-standard vocabulary of 'moral concern', 'moral standing', 'moral consideration', and so on. He was not deeply concerned with the question where the moral boundary should be drawn. Hence, it takes some work to connect his vocabulary to that of today's animal ethicists. Next up in this chapter, I will suggest a Kantian interpretation of the notion of 'moral concern'. I will then highlight three key elements of Kant's account of how we ought to treat others: first, his

[1] In Chap. 4, I will additionally argue that Kant's account of moral concern cannot be drawn directly from formulations of the Categorical Imperative. So the stereotype of Kantian moral concern as a quasi-algorithm is completely wrongheaded in my view.

N. D. Müller, *Kantianism for Animals*, The Palgrave Macmillan
Animal Ethics Series,
https://doi.org/10.1007/978-3-031-01930-2_2

doctrine of obligatory ends, which prescribes (among other things) that we promote the happiness of others; second, his account of moral concern as a reconciliation of duties 'of love' with duties 'of respect'; third, his division of our ethical duties towards others, which are put in terms of practical-emotional stances we ought to adopt or avoid vis à vis others, like 'sympathetic participation' and 'arrogance'. Before concluding, I will add some remarks on the *purpose* of Kant's account of moral concern. Kant differs from most of today's animal ethicists in that he does not view the primary purpose of ethics either in revising widespread moral beliefs and practices or in advising public policy. Kant's approach is rather that moral philosophy ought to *restore* and *refine* a moral standpoint ordinary people already endorse, but which is prone to corruption by our inclinations and self-serving rationalisations. I will explain how moral philosophy on this conception can still advance moral criticism and what other helpful uses it might have for animal ethicists. Overall, this chapter lays the foundation for the critical reflections and revisions in the next chapters.

To begin with, consider the notion of moral concern as it is used in contemporary animal ethics. It is a notion with several cognates: Whoever deserves[2] moral concern has 'moral status' (DeGrazia 1996; Warren 1997) or 'moral standing' (Frey 1988), is 'morally significant' (Pluhar 1995) or 'considerable' (Goodpaster 1978). What do we assert of an entity when we apply one of these predicates to it? First and foremost, the notion of moral concern is used for a moral demarcation: Who truly matters? In other words, the notion of moral concern and its cognates *pick out their subject* and *mark out its treatment as a matter of special moral relations or principles.* That which deserves moral concern ought to be at the centre of our moral reflections in a way that other things do not have to be. This is the core of the notion.

However, some authors mean something more specific by 'moral concern' or 'moral status'. The notion can refer to a special status that demands

---

[2] Talk of 'deserving' or 'being due' moral concern may seem suspicious to Kantians. After all, not all duties towards individuals are *owed* duties in Kant's view (see Sect. 2.4). For instance, there is a duty to be generous, but no one has a *right* or *claim* to be the recipient of generous gifts. However, to 'deserve' moral concern in the sense I propose here is not the same as being the object of owed duties. In the case of the duty to be generous, what we can be said to deserve is to be considered as a *possible* recipient, even if we have no claim to be the *actual* recipient. Stated generally, what we are *due* even in the case of meritorious duties is to be considered as possible patients under moral principles, even if those principles do not end up picking us out as actual patients.

a *specific* treatment for its bearer (over and above that of being particularly central in ethical reflections). Here, it can be useful to distinguish between *formal* and *substantive* senses of the terms. In a formal sense, to say that someone 'deserves moral concern' (is 'considerable', has 'moral standing', and so on) is merely to say that this individual *can* figure in moral relations or principles of a certain form. For instance, Warren explains that to have moral standing is "to be an entity towards which moral agents have, or can have, moral obligations" (Warren 1997, 3). What exactly those obligations demand is a separate question. Along similar lines, Korsgaard suggests that "'moral standing' is a stand-in, a kind of variable, for whatever it is that explains why we have obligations to the members of some group of entities" (Korsgaard 2018, 96). Thus, Korsgaard's notion of moral standing implies only *that* there are some obligations towards an individual (or that there is something about the individual which gives rise to obligations). But again, the notion does not specify what exactly those obligations demand of us.

By contrast, a *substantive* notion of moral concern already brings some 'moral baggage' with it, in the sense of moral content that makes the notion action-guiding to an extent. Take, for instance, the notion of 'moral status' employed by Jaworska and Tannenbaum: "[A]n animal may be said to have moral status if its suffering is at least somewhat morally bad, on account of this animal itself and regardless of the consequences for other beings" (Jaworska and Tannenbaum 2018). Hence, to say that some entity has moral status is already to say something substantive about how we ought to treat it: Its suffering ought to be avoided, other things being equal. Similarly, when Hoff (1983) claims that Kant denies animals have "moral standing", she is primarily concerned with his supposed indifference towards animal *well-being* (Hoff 1983, 67). To have moral standing, in Hoff's sense of the term, is for one's well-being to be a thing to be promoted (again, other things being equal). In this way, moral concern in a substantive sense is a notion implicitly tied to specific substantive moral principles about how to treat individuals. The difference between formal and substantive notions of moral concern is that substantive notions specify these principles, formal ones do not.

Among Kantians and Kant scholars, 'moral concern' and its cognates are not standardly used terms.[3] The notion of 'concern' does appear once

---

[3] One exception is Altman (2011), who uses 'moral concern', and almost all the cognates I have listed throughout his book. Another is Kain (2009), who uses 'moral status' throughout.

in a while as a non-technical expression (e.g. Wood 1998, 185; Svoboda 2012, 143, 2014, 320; Reath 2013, 208; Herman 2018, 174). Typically, however, Kant's readers do not give a very central role to notions like 'moral standing' or 'status'. They may even find them somewhat dubious and unclear (Sachs 2011; see also Hayward 1994, 130; Korsgaard 2018, 93ff.; Garthoff 2020). This is no coincidence. Kant's moral philosophy emphatically takes its starting point in the perspective of the agent, not in the perspective of those on the receiving end of actions. For Kant, moral philosophy answers the question "What ought I to do?" (CPR A805/B833)—not primarily "What ought to be done to me?". To begin thinking about ethical issues in terms of moral concern, from a Kantian point of view, is to put the cart before the horse. However, that does not entail that a Kantian cannot talk in terms of moral concern, but only that she must regard it as a function of moral agency, not vice versa. And when it comes to animal ethics, we do have good reasons to be interested in the recipients of actions, namely the animals: What ought to be done *to* them?[4] So what notion of moral concern should a Kantian endorse?

One might expect that for Kant, the term 'respect' takes the place now usually taken by 'moral concern' and its cognates. After all, Kant is widely associated with the view that all persons deserve respect. It would be natural to understand this simply as his way of expressing that persons *matter*. However, to simply equate 'respect' with 'moral concern' would be a mistake. Kant has several distinct notions of 'respect', and none of them map neatly onto the notion of 'moral concern' commonly used by animal and environmental ethicists today.

To see why the vocabulary is not congruent—but also to get a first glimpse into Kant's ethical universe—consider Kant's notions of 'respect'. The first and primary notion of respect at work in Kant's moral philosophy is the notion of 'respect for the moral law'. This term designates a feeling which enables the moral law to motivate action (G 4:400.29–33; CPrR 5:074.26–29). Of course, this notion of 'respect' cannot be very close to 'moral concern', simply because the object of this type of respect is the moral law, not a person.

---

[4] Increasingly, there are exceptions to this rule. Rowlands (2012) has investigated in what ways animals may be moral *subjects*, not merely *patients*, on the basis of his version of moral sentimentalism. Rutledge-Prior (2019) rejects Kantian morality precisely because it considers the capacity for morality to be exclusive to Kantian rational beings. Nonetheless, the bulk of animal ethics is about what humans may and ought to do *to* animals.

Secondly, respect for the moral law can be mediated through the example of a person, which is what Kant calls 'respect for persons' (G 4:401FN; CPrR 5:077.06–18; see Klimchuk 2003, 45–48). There are at least two species of respect for persons in Kant's writings.[5] One is 'respect' in the sense of a feeling of honour or praise for someone who embodies a good will by acting morally well. Using the term in this way, Kant is ready to claim that not all people deserve equal respect, since not all people act equally well (MM 6:448.17; MM 6:468.06–13; see Garcia 2012, 72–75). He also emphasises that "*respect* is always directed only to persons, never to things", where "things" is meant to include animals (CPrR 5:076.24).[6] But these statements do not express that scoundrels and animals do not deserve moral *concern* in today's vocabulary. Kant is talking about a feeling that responds to the moral worth of a good will, a kind of moral esteem or praise. Kant is quite simply saying that only moral agents are candidate objects for this kind of feeling. The other notion of 'respect for persons' we find Kant using is more egalitarian. It is a feeling appropriate to all persons, even scoundrels, in virtue of their *capacity* for morality, their *humanity* (G 4:436.02–06; see Garcia 2012, 81–83). Even though 'respect' in this sense takes a person for its object, we should not be too quick to equate the notion with that of 'moral concern'. After all, 'respect' here still refers to a *feeling* we find ourselves having for others; 'moral concern' and its cognates do not. There is however a difficult question whether the *requirement* of moral concern can be developed out of the conditions of respect for humanity—I will turn to this question in Chap. 4.

Third, Kant uses the notion of 'duties of respect' (MM 6:462.02–03). This is one of the two types of ethical duties we have towards others,

[5] Here, I leave out what Garcia calls 'political respect for persons' (Garcia 2012, 77–80), which amounts to treating others according to principles they could see as justified (Garcia 2012, 78). For Kant, this is not itself a species of respect, but rather a prerequisite of 'moral respect'(Garcia 2012, 80).

[6] Garcia discusses this passage under the heading of 'moral respect', which is the more egalitarian mode of respect for persons in virtue of the *capacity* for morality (Garcia 2012, 82). The context of the passage however suggests that Kant is concerned with 'respect' as honour or praise for someone who successfully observes the moral law. For instance, Kant asserts about the person whom we respect: "His example holds before me a law that strikes down my self-conceit when I compare it with my conduct, and I see *observance of that law and hence its practicability* proved before me in fact" (CPrR 5:077.06–09).

according to the *Doctrine of Virtue*. Here, 'respect' refers to a *practical* stance, not merely to a feeling (MM 6:449.23–30). To have respect in this sense is to adopt a maxim of not exalting ourselves above others (MM 6:449.32) and limiting our encroachment upon them out of a recognition that they are our equals in moral potential (MM 6:470.05–06). This sort of respect certainly forms a *part* of Kant's account of substantive moral concern—of how we ought to treat those who matter morally. However, 'respect' does not *fully* capture the way in which we ought to treat others, since there is also another kind of ethical duty towards others called *duties of love* (MM 6:448.07; MM 6:449.17–22). Once again, Kant's 'respect' does not equal 'moral concern'.

What, then, *does* correspond to 'moral concern' in Kant's system? To get the analysis off the ground, we should understand 'moral concern' as only one term in a set of interrelated quasi-technical terms: *Moral concern* is the appropriate attitude towards *moral patients*. *Moral patients* are all beings towards whom there are *duties*.

The Kantian way to lend meaning to these terms is to give primacy to the bottom row of Table 2.1 and work our way upwards. 'Duty towards X' is the only notion in the table that also appears in Kant's own writings. The rest can be developed from it. We can develop *formal* notions of patienthood and concern in this table if we leave open which exact duties are at issue. Just as well, however, can we fill in specific duties in the bottom row to yield a *substantive* notion of concern on top.

Moral patients, accordingly, should be understood to be those towards whom (some specific) Kantian duties are directed.[7] Moral concern is the appropriate attitude towards individuals specifically insofar as they are moral patients. Hence, moral concern is the attitude that is appropriate vis

Table 2.1 Terms related to moral concern

	Concern-related terms
Appropriate attitude	Moral concern
Individual	Moral patient
Necessitation	Duty towards X

[7] This is a broader notion of moral patienthood than Regan employs. According to my notion, most adult human beings are moral agents *and* moral patients—they have duties and there are duties towards them. By contrast, Regan reserves the notion of moral patienthood for beings *incapable* of having duties (Regan 2004, 152).

à vis those towards whom we have duties. Among other things, we can then characterise a formal notion of moral concern 'Kantian-style' as the attitude of *recognising* that one has duties towards some individual and of *resolve* to do as one's duty towards them demands (assuming that this is the appropriate attitude to take vis à vis those to whom we have duties).

Of course, this understanding of 'moral concern' renders the exegetical question trivial *whether* Kant grants animals moral concern. He clearly does not, since he denies that there are duties towards animals. To Kantians, this may seem somewhat dysphemistic. To claim that Kant 'denies animals moral concern' makes it sound as if he allowed *just any* treatment of animals, no matter how cruel. This he does not—he is opposed to the cruel and ungrateful treatment of animals (MM 6:443.10–16; see Chap. 3). So it is worth keeping in mind that being the object of moral concern, to *matter* morally, is not strictly the same thing as *being protected by certain duties*. One can be protected without mattering for one's own sake.

Some in the literature would tend to understand moral concern differently. One option is to use 'moral concern' to designate a stance of sympathy and gratitude (which Kant asks us to adopt vis à vis animals). However, this use of the label is somewhat ad hoc.[8] Just as we have duties of sympathy and gratitude 'regarding' animals, we have duties of aesthetic appreciation 'regarding' plants and lifeless nature, and still other duties 'regarding' God (MM 6:443.27–31). Why should we single out objects of sympathy and gratitude, but not those of aesthetic appreciation? More consistent, but still unattractive, would it be to use 'moral concern' as a label designating an attitude towards anything 'regarding' which we have duties. This label would apply to flatly anything in this world and beyond, from plants and crystallisations all the way up to God Almighty (since there are Kantian duties 'regarding' all these entities, MM 6:443.02–32; see Chap. 3). But the label 'moral concern' is supposed to designate some *special* moral significance that not all entities have. So I will use 'moral

---

[8] Svoboda makes a similar move when he claims that it constitutes "a kind of moral consideration" (Svoboda 2012 161) that "Kant's account of duties regarding non-human natural entities gives human beings good moral reason both to benefit animals and flora and to abstain from causing them unnecessary harm" (ibid.). But this is an overstatement of Kant's position, as I will explain in Sect. 3.2. Kant does not and cannot demand that we avoid harming animals—or that we benefit them—across the board. He can only demand this *insofar as doing so cultivates a natural capacity serviceable to morality*. But what is good for animals is not always good for our capacities, and vice versa.

concern' in one of the received ways (Warren 1997, 3): as a label denoting the appropriate attitude to beings *towards* whom we have duties, not just *regarding*.[9]

Finally, there may be another worry about the vocabulary proposed here: If moral concern is analysable in terms of our duties, why talk in terms of moral concern at all? Why not cut out the middleman and simply talk about our duties towards animals? Indeed, much of the discussion in the coming chapters will be in terms of our duties. Still, the vocabulary of 'moral concern' and its cognates is useful for three reasons: First, it connects the common professional language of animal ethicists to that of Kant scholars. Second, it enables us to talk in terms of moral attitudes, which will be useful when discussing the role of respect for humanity (Chap. 4) and whether the requirement of concern for others can be developed out of it. Third, the vocabulary of attitudes emphasises an aspect of Kantian duties which is often downplayed or overlooked, namely their attachment to a feeling, caring, other-oriented human being. Hence, though much of the present project revolves around our duties, I will also continue to make use of the vocabulary of 'moral concern'.

Towards whom, then, do we have duties? Kant never states an explicit account of the boundary of moral concern. What he does provide, however, are some *necessary conditions* that must be met in order for duties to obtain towards someone:

> Judging according to mere reason, a human being has no duty other than merely to a human being (himself or another); for his duty to any subject is moral necessitation by this subject's will. The necessitating (obligating) subject must therefore, *first*, be a person, and, *secondly*, this person must be given as an object of experience. (MM 6:442.08–13)

The first condition, being capable of 'necessitating' or 'constraining'[10] others, is what excludes animals—as well as plants and lifeless nature, for

---

[9] This use is also close to Hayward's preferred terminology, which equates 'standing' with the 'capacity to bear rights' (Hayward 1994, 141). However, for Kant not all duties correspond to rights (MM 6:383.05–08). For this reason, I prefer to focus on duties rather than rights.

[10] 'Constraint' is Gregor's translation (Gregor 1996). Kant's German term is "*Nöthigung*" (MM 6:442.08), which more straightforwardly translates to 'necessitation' (Gregor, Timmermann & Grenberg forthcoming). From a philosophical standpoint, there is something to be said in favour of setting apart Kant's term '*Nöthigung*' in the sense of an

that matter (MM 6:442.28–31). The second condition, being an object of experience, is what excludes God and angels (MM 6:442.31–33).

Kant does not make it explicit what interpersonal 'necessitation' consists in. A more detailed discussion of this issue will have to wait until Chap. 5. In any case, however, it is fair to assume that Kant has a relation in mind which can only obtain between beings capable of morality. Only a will capable of 'constraining' itself can 'constrain' others. So Kant's criteria imply that we can have duties only towards finite rational beings capable of morality, and human beings are the only such creatures we know (MM 6:442.16–18).

Kant's first condition raises the question whether we have duties towards literally all members of the human species, including those who are not capable of morality (Dombrowski 1997, 30; Kain 2009, 61). It would seem harsh of Kant to deny that we have any duties, say, towards small infants and certain people with disabilities. Kant here faces a *modus tollens* argument commonly known in animal ethics as the 'argument from species overlap': If we have no duties towards animals, there are also no duties towards certain human beings; but we do have duties towards all human beings; therefore we have some duties towards animals (Horta 2014, 145; see also Dombrowski 1997, 1f.). Just as well known, however, are the standard responses to the argument: emphasising the importance of potentiality, similarity, or membership in a kind (Frey 1977, 188; Cohen 2001, 37). If we can argue, for instance, that Kantian moral concern hinges not on an *actual* necessitating or constraining activity of the will, but rather on the *predisposition* to become a being with a constraining will, his view does not have to conflict with our commitment to the moral status of all human beings. As Kain has shown in great detail, Kant's biological and psychological views allow for a case along these lines (Kain 2009). However, as Kain also points out, such a case would have to rely on a species essentialism that is incompatible with an evolutionary perspective (Kain 2009, 101). Only if all species members have an essential potential in common, and only if human essence in particular includes the potential to become capable of morality, does the argument from species overlap let

---

interpersonal relation (as in MM 6:442.10) from his usual use of '*Nöthigung*' in the sense of a person's necessitation by the moral law (e.g. in G 4:413.04; G 4:417.05; G 4:439.31; CPrR 5:032.24–25; CPrR 5:082.10–11; CPrR 5:117.18–19; MM 6:379.15; MM 6:401.33; MM 6:437.32; MM 6:481.34; MM 6:487.18). The two are not identical. However, this difference need not be made explicit in the course of translation. We may as well keep in mind that '*Nöthigung*', always translated as 'necessitation', is ambiguous.

Kant off the hook. So even though the historical Kant believed in the moral status of literally all human beings, for today's Kantians his supporting argument creates greater problems than it solves. In general, this is yet another reason to be interested in a version of Kantianism that manages to include beings incapable of morality.

What this section has argued is that we can and should understand Kantian moral concern—what it means to 'matter' in Kant's ethical universe—as a function of duties. Moral concern is the appropriate attitude towards moral patients, and moral patients are those towards whom we have duties. Kant believes that all and only moral agents matter in this sense. Before delving into the question how we might disagree, let me illustrate the treatment human beings receive in Kant's system.

2.2   Kant's Taxonomy of Duties

Having some grasp of the beings towards whom we have duties, what actual duties do we have? Kant has an interesting way of ordering our duties, based on distinctions that are no longer as familiar as they were to readers of European philosophy in the eighteenth century. In particular, Kant follows the tradition in distinguishing between perfect versus imperfect duties, duties towards self versus others, duties of right versus virtue, and within duties of virtue to others, between duties of love versus respect.[11] He however offers his own version of each distinction, and each revolves around a property of our duties. Hence, we say a great deal about the nature of some specific duty when we categorise it as, say, an imperfect duty of love towards others.

To see Kant's distinctions in action, consider the four examples of duties he mentions in the *Groundwork*:

(1) Not to commit prudential suicide (G 4:397.33; G 4:421.24)
(2) Not to give false promises (G 4:422.15)
(3) To develop our natural talents (G 4:422.27)
(4) To be beneficent (G 4:398.08; G 4:423.17)

---

[11] These are not all of Kant's distinctions. He also draws further distinctions, such as the distinction between duties towards self as a natural being vs. purely as a moral being (MM 6:421.07–08; MM 6:428.28–29). I will use this distinction below in Chap. 9 but stick to the more basic distinctions in the exposition here.

Even if one has not read any Kant before, one can recognise some systematicity in this list. The first two are put in negative terms, the latter two in positive terms. This corresponds to Kant's distinction between perfect and imperfect duties. The crucial property of perfect duties is that they do not allow for any exceptions (G 4:421FN). Whenever we *can* observe a perfect duty (e.g. not to give a false promise), we *must*. By contrast, imperfect duties allow for observance in many different situations and in many different ways, so that we must choose when and how to observe them. For example, there are many opportunities to cultivate our natural talents, and we must judge which of them we should actually take. In the *Groundwork*, Kant also provides a slightly more technical account of the perfect-imperfect distinction: Perfect duties are those we violate when we adopt maxims that cannot be universalised. Imperfect duties, by contrast, are those which we violate by adopting maxims which we could universalise, but could not *will* in their universalised form (G 4:424.01–14; see *Mongrovius* 29:610).

What we can also see from Kant's four examples is that the duties not to commit prudential suicide and to develop our natural talents have directly to do with the agent herself, while the duties not to give false promises and to be beneficent have more directly to do with her treatment of others. This corresponds to Kant's distinction between duties to self and others. The existence of duties to self is a crucial—and in comparison to today's dominant approaches to animal ethics, a fairly unique—aspect of Kant's outlook on morality: that how we treat ourselves matters morally as much as how we treat others. Morality is not just a matter of respecting another's boundaries and being beneficent, but it is also a matter of comporting oneself with the right stance towards oneself.

All of that said, the *Groundwork* is not intended as a full account of what all our ethical duties demand of us (see Timmermann 2007a, xi). That is not the *Groundwork*'s task. Its task is to establish the supreme moral principle, the Categorical Imperative, based on a conception of the good will Kant presumes we share (see Wood 2007, 53; Trampota 2013, 145). The purpose of the Categorical Imperative itself is not to state a particular duty. We may have a duty to obey the Categorical Imperative, to be sure, but it is not obvious that this way of putting our duty is itself action-guiding. It may be more like a duty 'to do the right thing'—a duty we may have, but which does not *substantively* tell us what we ought to do (for more on this see Chap. 4).

Kant's most developed account of what we ought to do comes in what is arguably his principal work in moral philosophy (Trampota 2013, 141), the *Metaphysics of Morals* of 1797. In its second half, the *Doctrine of Virtue*, he aims to provide a *taxonomy* of our moral duties, that is, a system of distinctions. Contained in this taxonomy are both distinctions already mentioned, between duties to self and others, and between perfect and imperfect duties.[12]

Another interesting aspect of Kant's moral philosophy is that it addresses not just the rightness or wrongness of mere acts, but also the moral quality of motives. For both, Kant has a category for duties: 'Strict' duties, also called 'duties of right', prescribe mere acts irrespective of motive. 'Wide' duties or 'duties of virtue' prescribe that we adopt certain *ends*. The main characteristic of 'wide' duties is that their observance allows for a certain "latitude" (MM 6:390.06–09). What Kant means, however, is not that we can pick and choose *whether* to observe our wide duties (MM 6:390.09–12). Since they are duties, we ought always to observe them whenever they obtain. Kant rather means to say that wide duties prescribe that we adopt certain ends or maxims, rather than that we perform certain acts (MM 6:388.32–33). But maxims or ends are, by their nature, general and can get in each other's way. Kant's own example is that a maxim of charity towards all human beings may be restricted by a maxim of parental love (MM 6:390.12). So the distinguishing feature of 'wide' duties is that they can restrict each other, even though we must still not make any exceptions for the sake of our inclinations.

---

[12] More precisely, Kant now uses two perfect-imperfect distinctions (Freiin von Villiez 2015, 1757; Rühl 2015, 1753). One, which can be found throughout the main text of the *Doctrine of Virtue*, is similar to the old *Groundwork* distinction, according to which perfect duties do not allow for any exceptions, while imperfect duties do. However, the reason why exceptions are permitted is not that inclination may take precedence (as the *Groundwork* seemed to imply), but that imperfect duties can be observed in many different situations. For instance, Kant asserts that we have an imperfect duty towards self to positively develop our natural talents (MM 6:444.18–20). That this duty is imperfect does not imply that we may be lazy whenever we feel like it. It rather implies that there are many natural talents, and many situations in which to develop them, so that we must choose when and how to observe this duty. The determining factors for this choice are not our inclinations, but rather our other perfect and imperfect duties. In the introduction to the *Metaphysics of Morals*, however, Kant uses the same terms differently. Here, he equates perfect duties with 'strict' duties, and imperfect duties with 'wide' duties (MM 6:390.14–18). Ethics in the narrow sense is concerned with 'imperfect' or 'wide' duties, while the law is concerned with 'perfect' or 'strict' duties (MM 6:388.32–33).

To animal ethicists who do not specialise in Kant scholarship, the notion of a wide duty should be particularly noteworthy in two respects: First, Kant's moral philosophy is not completely negative and procedural, in the sense of only giving necessary moral conditions for our maxims (an impression one might have gotten from Rawls's influential 'four-step CI procedure', Rawls 2000, 167ff.). In the vocabulary of wide duties, Kant positively states *ends* that we ought to adopt. Secondly, Kant's moral philosophy is not completely absolutist, in the sense of prescribing specific duties that must be obeyed without regard to the context of the particular situation. In principle, we should always consider any wide duty in context with *all* other duties. Because this is impossible to do in practice, Kant does not answer first-order normative questions in ethics with a strict 'yes' or 'no'. Rather, he highlights certain considerations (see Wood 2007, 48f.) and then provokes his readers to judge for themselves how their duties interact by means of 'casuistical questions' at the end of many sections of the *Doctrine of Virtue* (MM 6:423.17–424.08; MM 6:426.01–32; MM 6:428.01–26; MM 6:431.16–34; MM 6:433.06–434.19; MM 6:437.03–26; MM 6:454.01–28; MM 6:458.01–19).

Besides the perfect-imperfect contrast, the distinction between *duties to self* and *duties to others* is the central ordering principle of the *Doctrine of Virtue*. So the 'directionality' of duties—their character of being directed 'towards' someone—takes a central place. Unfortunately, just as Kant does not provide a positive account of moral patienthood, he does not provide a positive account of the directionality of our duties. What is clear, in any case, is that our duties to self and others prescribe different ends. Kant calls these the 'ends that are also duties' (MM 6:382.06–07). Our overarching duty to ourselves is *to promote our own moral perfection* (MM 6:391.29.; MM 6:398). 'Moral perfection' here denotes moral goodness, but not only that. It also refers more generally to being a good observer of duties, to act in a way that is appropriate to a subject capable of morality. This includes keeping ourselves in good moral shape, for instance by avoiding overindulgence in drugs which make it harder to determine our actions freely (MM 6:427.12–15). It also includes acting in a way that acknowledges our fundamental moral equality to all other rational beings, which proscribes being servile to others (MM 6:434.32–435.05). For readers today, the word 'integrity' might more intuitively describe what Kant means by 'perfection'.

Duties towards others, by contrast, can be subsumed under the obligatory end of *promoting the happiness of others* (MM 6:393.10; MM

6:398)—this will be the topic of the next section.[13] Before exploring this issue further, we can already see that Kant would *not* think of substantive moral concern as one uniform attitude which we ought to have towards both ourselves and others. Regarding others, moral concern consists in such stances as practical benevolence, gratitude, and sympathetic participation (though it must be properly restricted by respect, see Sect. 2.4 below). These are appropriate attitudes to beings whose happiness it is our duty to promote. By contrast, moral concern for oneself has little to do with promoting one's own happiness—it is not prudence or self-love by any stretch. Rather, it is the appropriate attitude towards the being whose moral perfection we ought to promote (ourselves). We can take this to be an attitude of moral aspiration, but plausibly also of a certain moral rigour or discipline. In Kant's own words, he asks the human being "to be of a *robust* and *cheerful* mind (*animus strenuus et hilaris*) in observing its duties" (MM 6:484.21–22). I should add that we also have what Kant calls an 'indirect' duty to secure our own happiness, since being severely deprived makes it more tempting for us to violate our duties (MM 6:388.26–28). But in general, there is no duty to promote our own happiness—that is other people's task.

2.3   OTHERS' HAPPINESS AS AN OBLIGATORY END

Kant is often portrayed as a philosopher inimical to happiness, or at least uninterested in it. Indeed, Kant did hold that an action's *moral worth* does not depend on whether it produces happiness, but on whether it springs from a good will (GMS 4:393.05–24). However, to say that happiness does not determine moral worth is not to deny it all value. Happiness is valuable for Kant in the sense that it is *something we ought to bring about in others*. Kant's way of expressing this is to say that the happiness of others is an "end that is at the same time one's duty" (MM 6:393.11; MM 6:398), which I will call an 'obligatory end' for short. To be clear, our duty is not to *like* another's happiness as a matter of passive affect (MM 6:402.22–25), which we cannot force ourselves to do. Nor is it simply to *wish* that others achieve happiness without taking any action (MM 6:452.01–03). Rather, our duty is to adopt a maxim of *beneficence*, of

---

[13] At this point, I skip over some taxonomic problems, particularly the difficult question how 'duties of respect' can be duties to others, yet not follow from the obligatory end of the happiness of others (Fahmy 2013). I will return to this issue in Sect. 2.4 and later in 6.1.

aiming to bring about another's happiness by means of our actions (MM 6:452.04–05; see Moran 2017, 322). While 'beneficence' denotes the successful act of promoting another's happiness (MM 6:453.02; see Moran 2016, 343), Kant calls the *stance* we ought to take towards others' 'practical benevolence' (MM 6:452.04).

At first sight, this moral instruction seems very coarse-grained—as if others had a certain simple property, *happiness*, which we must strive to intensify. However, this obligatory end also admits of a more fine-grained description if we take a closer look at what 'happiness' is according to Kant.

First, happiness consists in well-being that can be qualitatively *physical* as well as qualitatively *moral* (Kang 2015, 14; see Zöller 2013, 23). By 'physical well-being', Kant means the greatest possible amount of pleasure (CPJ 5:208.22–25; CPrR 5:117.25–26; B834/A806; CPrR 5:073.09–11; G 4:399.12; CPrR 5:022.17–19). For instance, in the third *Critique*, Kant calls happiness "the greatest sum (regarding both amount and duration) of life's pleasantness" (CPJ 5:208.22–25). On the other hand, however, Kant also acknowledges that human beings feel a distinct kind of pleasure upon following the moral law (MM 6:378.13–14), "a state of peace of soul and contentment" (MM 6:377.21), also simply called "moral pleasure" (MM 6:391.12). Hence, although Kant's conception of happiness is hedonistic (happiness is a function of hedonic states), he accepts that there is a kind of hedonic state we can only experience because we are capable of morality. Physical and moral well-being do not represent two distinct kinds of happiness, but they represent qualitatively different kinds of hedonic states that both contribute to the happiness of a human being overall. For this reason, we human beings are happy only if we are content *both* with our natural state *and* with our own moral conduct. Conversely, physical pain is a threat to happiness, but so is a bad conscience or self-contempt.

Secondly, happiness is something we *strive for* as a matter of inclination. This is the *practical* side of Kant's conception of human happiness (see Kang 2015, 24–27). Kant repeatedly characterises happiness as an *end* of human beings (G 4:415.28–33; CPrR 5:124.21–25) and as that which "everyone unavoidably already wants by himself" (MM 6:386.03–04). Kant also emphatically calls a person's happiness the condition under which "everything goes according to his wish and will" (CPrR 5:124.22–24; see MM 6:480.21–22). This practical characterisation of happiness does not contradict the hedonic one, but it complements and specifies it.

Happiness is a matter of positive hedonic states, but our *pursuit* of it is structured by practical reason.

The claim that we naturally seek to promote our own happiness plays an important role in Kant's ethics: "So, when what counts is happiness, as an end that it is my duty to effect, it must be the happiness of *other* human beings, *whose* (permissible) *end I thereby also* make *my own*" (MM 6:388.05–08). Thus, Kant asks us to adopt *another's end*. To be certain, Kant here only means to assert that we ought to adopt the end of others *de re*, not *de dicto*. That is to say, we do not have to adopt *whatever* ends others might happen to set for themselves. Rather, we ought to adopt the end which other human beings can be presumed to pursue, which is their happiness. Even if a human being were brainwashed into pursuing some other ultimate end, what we should make our end is still their happiness. However, an agent's self-chosen ends and inclinations are nevertheless crucial for beneficence. In perhaps a slightly hyperbolic remark, Kant claims about other human beings: "What they may count as belonging to their happiness is left to their own judgement" (MM 6:388.08–09). Kant does not mean to say that we can will it so that any object of choice makes us happy—we cannot decide that going hungry should make us happy. What we can decide, however, is by what *means* we pursue our happiness. And when it comes to beneficence, Kant's picture is that others' ends and inclinations should be our principal guideposts. As he puts it in the *Groundwork*, "the ends of a subject who is an end in itself must as far as possible be also *my* ends" (G 4:430.24–27). And in the *Doctrine of Virtue*: "The duty of love of one's neighbour can therefore also be expressed thus: it is the duty to make the *ends* of others my own" (MM 6:340.03–05). And later again: "I cannot be beneficent to anyone according to *my* concepts of happiness (except for children during their minority or the mentally disturbed), but only according to the concepts of *him* whom I would like to render a benefit by urging a gift upon him" (MM 6:454.18–21).[14] Hence, insofar as others are competent pursuers of their own happiness, our primary task is to assist them in their own self-chosen endeavours. This gives Kant's account of beneficence an anti-paternalistic flavour.

---

[14] Of course, this remark in particular raises the question why Kant's emphasis on the patient's own ends and inclinations should transfer to our treatment of animals, even granted that we have a duty to promote their happiness. After all, if Kant already specifies that we may paternalise children and cognitively atypical people, why not animals? I address this difficulty in Sect. 6.2 below.

How does reason involve itself in the pursuit of happiness? On this matter, Kant is quite explicit: Reason has a "commission from the side of [a human being's] sensibility which it cannot refuse" (CPrR 5:061.26–27). It is the 'commission' to "form maxims with a view to happiness" (CPrR 5:061.28–29)—that is to say, to choose the means to the preconceived end of happiness. So instrumental practical reason only 'sets ends' in a very restricted sense. It cannot set any ends *ex nihilo*, as perhaps a more existentialist view might have it. Instrumental practical reason is purely in the business of choosing *means* to happiness, even if these means are themselves intermediary *ends*.

When Kant invokes this picture, he is usually concerned with arguing that reason is not *restricted* to the task of merely choosing means to a preordained end—that reason can by itself be practical. Take his argument in the second *Critique*: If there is a 'higher' faculty of desire, a faculty of desire that *requires* reason, then there must be an end that takes its origin in reason alone, not the senses (CPrR 5:062.01–07). Otherwise, reason would only be in the business of reordering the materials provided to it by sensibility. Similarly, in the *Groundwork*, Kant remarks that reason is quite inept at securing happiness, or at least less apt than instinct, and that therefore securing happiness cannot be reason's true purpose (G 4:396.14–24). Still, both these arguments presuppose that instrumental practical reason really *does* involve itself in our pursuit of happiness, inept as it may be.

Inherent in Kant's conception of reason's involvement in the pursuit of happiness is the idea of a *system* or *hierarchy* of ends and inclinations. An order is necessary, for one thing, because our various inclinations and ends can conflict, and reason has to be the arbiter. As Kant puts it in the *Religion*: "*Considered in themselves* natural inclinations are *good* […]; we must rather only curb them, so that they will not wear each other out but will instead be harmonised into a whole called happiness" (Rel 6:058.01–06). Another kind of hierarchy is established by instrumental-rational considerations. Our non-moral ends are themselves practical means to further ends, and all our non-moral ends can ultimately be subsumed under the end of happiness, which Kant calls our "whole" end for this reason (CPrR 5:124.24).

The idea that reason orders and harmonises our pursuit of happiness has important ramifications: If our duty is to promote the happiness of others, and if we are to use their own ends and inclinations as guideposts, then evidently we do not have to promote another's *next best* inclination or end. Rather, we should employ our own capacities of practical reason to judge, as best we can, which of the other person's ends or inclinations we should promote. We must regard their pursuit of happiness as a systematic union and do what best promotes the higher-up ends and inclinations. In this way, we can derive quite specific instructions from Kant's doctrine of obligatory ends.

What I hope the discussion in this section conveys to animal ethicists is that, first, Kant has quite intricate and systematic views on happiness, and he gives the promotion of happiness an important place in ethics. Secondly, however, Kant's conception of the human pursuit of happiness operates in terms of rational capacities. This will pose some difficulties when we try to modify the framework and include animals in it—I will return to these difficulties in Chap. 6.

2.4   PRACTICAL LOVE AND RESPECT FOR OTHERS

As we have just seen, we can derive very general and very specific ethical instructions from Kant's doctrine of obligatory ends. However, Kant himself devotes most of his attention in the *Doctrine of Virtue* to duties at an in-between level of generality. Among our duties towards others, he distinguishes two types and then goes on to characterise what we might call *practical-emotional stances* we ought to take (or avoid to take) towards others, such as *gratitude* (MM 6: 454.30), *envy*, *modesty*, and *malicious glee* (MM 6:458.23–24). These are *stances* in the sense that they are attitudes we voluntarily take towards others, and which we would be capable of avoiding. They are *practical* in the sense that they bear a connection to action rather than being entirely contemplative. And they are *emotional* in the sense that they bear an intimate connection to feelings we find ourselves having about others and ourselves.

Kant's "division" (MM 6:448.08) of duties towards others is effectively a taxonomy of practical-emotional stances, either to be adopted or to be avoided. The chief distinction in this taxonomy is between duties of love and duties of respect (MM 6.118.10 15). Duties of love ask us to adopt practical-emotional stances that befit the promotion of the happiness of others—Kant names beneficence, gratitude, and sympathetic participation in another's weal and woe. Duties of love are all about practical love, that is the active promotion of another's happiness. By contrast, duties of respect put certain restrictions on *how* we should go about pursuing this obligatory end. Other human beings stand under the moral law and therefore share with all others the fundamental potential for morality (no matter how badly they actually act). We should recognise, and act in accordance with, this fundamental moral equality. In particular, this implies that we should not exalt ourselves above others (MM 6:449.32; see Sensen 2013, 352), neither by being arrogant or contemptuous towards them, nor by being overbearingly beneficent without regard for their self-esteem. As Kant writes:

> Thus we will recognize our obligation to be beneficent towards someone poor; but since this favour yet also involves dependence of his weal upon my generosity, which after all demeans the other, it is our duty to spare the recipient this humiliation and to preserve his respect for himself by our comportment, representing this beneficence either as merely what is owed or as a slight labour of love. (MM 6:448.22–449.02)

Kant's point is not that there is anything inherently humiliating about benefitting from another's help. It is rather that generosity also burdens the beneficiary with a duty to be grateful (Moran 2017, 314), as well as a social expectation to pay back what was given. As the *Collins* lecture notes report Kant saying:

> A debtor is at all times under the constraint of having to treat the person he is obliged to with politeness and flattery; [...] But he who pays promptly for everything can act freely, and nobody will hamper him in doing so. (*Collins* 27:341f.)

So the real threat to moral self-esteem is not beneficence in itself, but the social expectations which it places on the beneficiary. We fail to treat others as equally free rational beings if we burden them with too many duties of gratitude and politeness. So proper respect for others should constrain the extent to which we are beneficent to others and the way in which we present our own beneficence ("as merely what is owed or as a slight labour of love", MM 6:448.26–449.01).

The interplay between these two kinds of duties is crucial for the way in which Kant's ethical system works in application. In several different ways, duties of love and duties of respect are mutually opposing forces, and our moral treatment of others is a matter of balancing or reconciling their contrary demands. Kant draws three principal distinctions between the two duty-types:

First, and most emphatically, Kant draws a *normative* distinction: Fulfilling some of our duties puts the patient under a reciprocal obligation (MM 6:448.10–12). In some instances, the patient acquires an obligation towards the benefactor to be grateful (MM 6:454.31–32). Such obligations only arise in the case of duties of love, not duties of respect. That is, we have a duty to be grateful for what others do to us with love, but not for what they do to us with respect. Kant also expresses this normative difference by designating duties of love as 'meritorious' duties and duties of respect as 'owed' duties (MM 6:448.13–14).

To ward off a misunderstanding, we should not confuse the *meritorious* with the *supererogatory* (Timmermann 2006, 22; Vogt 2009, 221; Schönecker 2013, 313). Our duties of love are meritorious, but they have an obligating character just as much as owed duties do. To pick an example: It is an obligation, not supererogatory, to be beneficent (MM 6:452.26–30). If we fail to observe this duty, we have reason for self-reproach, and others may have reason to morally object to our conduct. And still, whoever happens to be our beneficiary acquires a duty to be grateful. Conversely, those who do not happen to have benefitted have no grounds to object (so long as we were sufficiently beneficent), since there is no claim to be the beneficiary of any particular act of beneficence. In this way, duties of love do not correspond to any particular claim on the part of the patient, but duties of respect do.

Secondly, Kant draws a *phenomenological* distinction: Our observance of some duties is accompanied by a feeling of love, for other duties, it is a feeling of respect for others (MM 6:448.14–15).[15] Both of these feelings are therefore associated with Kantian moral concern. While Kant himself stresses the feelings we have *for others*, we could plausibly claim that the duty-types are also accompanied by different feelings *about ourselves*, or about the *relation* between ourselves and the patient. When we act from a duty of respect, we feel that *we owe* someone some treatment. By contrast,

---

[15] Schönecker insists that duties of love and respect cannot be distinguished by their accompanying feelings (Schönecker 2013, 314), *pace* earlier readers (Gregor 1963; Forkl 2001). To my mind, Kant's statement on the matter leaves little room for doubt: "*Love* and *respect* are the feelings that accompany the carrying out of these duties" (MM 6:448.14–15). Schönecker's main argument is that Kant asserts that we feel respect for our benefactors when we are grateful, even though the duty of gratitude is a duty of love (MM 6:454.32–33). To be fully precise, however, Kant only asserts that the *judgement* that another has rendered us a benefit is accompanied by respect (MM 6:454.32). But our fulfilment of the *duty* to act in a way befitting gratitude can still be accompanied by a feeling of love.

when we act from a duty of love, we feel that *we grant* the beneficiary something. Hence, we take ourselves to be in a very different position vis à vis the moral patient.

As we can see, moral life according to Kant has an important *emotional* dimension.[16] Our fulfilment of duties towards others is necessarily accompanied by the characteristic feelings of love and respect. On this note, consider also that Kant emphasises the distinct feeling of respect *for the moral law* which plays a crucial role in any moral motivation according to Kant (e.g. G 4:400.18–19; G 4:401FN; CPrR 5:081.10–13). Conscience, too, is connected to feelings: "No human being is altogether without moral feeling; for complete lack of receptivity to this sensation would render him morally dead" (MM 6:400.09–11). And even then, we have not listed all the emotions Kant acknowledges to play an important role in our moral lives (Schönecker 2013, 326). Built into Kant's conception of moral concern are also the more contingent feelings of "rejoicing with others and feeling pity for them" (MM 6:456.20), gratitude (MM 6:454.03–04), "gratification in the happiness (well-being) of others" (MM 6:452.27), as well as the emotional aspect of practical-emotional stances discussed by Kant, such as the aforementioned "envy, ingratitude, and malicious glee" (MM 6:458.23f). All of this goes to show that the stereotype of Kant as a philosopher dismissive of feelings is unwarranted.

Third, Kant draws a *substantive* distinction: Our duties of love demand something else than our duties of respect. Duties of love demand that we adopt and observe a maxim of practical benevolence towards others (MM 6:449.17–22; see Rinne 2018, 132). Duties of respect, by contrast, demand that we adopt a maxim of limiting our self-esteem in view of others' dignity (MM 6:449.23–30).[17] We ought to acknowledge others as our moral equals, as beings who, like ourselves, have a potential for moral goodness that nothing else in the world has. Kant illustrates the difference with the metaphor of an 'attractive force' (love) and a 'repellent force' (respect) (MM 6:470.04–05). What Kant is getting at is that some of our

---

[16] I mention this, of course, because the impression that Kant denigrates the emotions in moral life is very influential. There seems to be a consensus among Kant's readers, however, that the emotions have an important role to play, even though they do not account for an action's moral worth. For a more detailed discussion, see Hay (2013, 56–62) and Rinne (2018).

[17] Of course, this complicates things as soon as we attempt to adopt this maxim towards animals, who (we may assume) do not have the 'dignity' characteristic only of moral agents. I consider this difficulty in Chap. 6 below.

duties encourage getting involved in others' affairs, while other duties demand that we do not encroach upon others (Sensen 2013, 344).

As central as they are to Kant's account of moral concern for others, duties of respect also pose some problems for Kant's taxonomy. How can duties of respect count as duties of virtue, which are supposed to prescribe a positive end, when their demand is essentially negative (Fahmy 2013, 729)? How can they count as duties towards others, if they do not demand that we promote the happiness of others as an obligatory end, but instead that we *limit* our beneficence (Fahmy 2013, 726f.)? Kant seems to think that the recognition of another's equal humanity puts certain normative constraints on our relations to others quite independently from the two obligatory ends. Frankly, this is an area in which Kant's taxonomy is not very orderly. Part of my argument in Chap. 6 will rest on a purposeful recategorisation of duties of respect which removes the confusion and makes it clearer why we ought not to exalt ourselves above others and why this requirement can restrict our beneficence. For the moment, what I hope animal ethicists can gain from this discussion is that Kant's account of our duties to others revolves around the reconciliation of duties of love with duties of respect (even if the origin of the latter is admittedly somewhat obscure).

As Kant puts it, duties of love and respect are "accessorily connected" (MM 6:447.22).[18] That is, some duties obtain *only because* certain others obtain, such that "one duty [...] accedes, as it were, to another" (Schönecker 2013, 322). This order results from the way moral agents cognise and act on the moral law. Kant asserts that all our duties "are really always united with each other according to the law in a single duty, yet only in such a way that now one duty, now the other constitutes the principle in the subject, such that one duty is joined to the other accessorily" (MM 6:448.19–22).[19] The picture Kant is sketching here is that of a net of interconnected duties, each representing some aspect of what we ought to do overall. Were we to formulate the "single duty" in which all our duties are united, it would either be an infinite conjunct of duties, which

---

[18] For MM 6:448.19–22, I use Schönecker's translation (Schönecker 2013, 319) because I agree with him that the translation "as accessory" (Gregor 1996) can be misleading. The same is true, by extension, for the translation "as an accessory" (Timmermann forthcoming).

[19] Some readers take Kant to say that it is our *feelings* of love and respect that are "accessorily connected" but are puzzled by this claim (Schönecker 2013, 318). I agree with Schönecker that Kant's passage is more straightforward if we read *duties* as connected in this way, not their accompanying feelings.

we cannot cognise, or it would simply be a duty to observe the Categorical Imperative, which does not give specific action-guidance. Our best option is to cognise some specific duties at a time. Hence, any statement of a specific duty gives only an incomplete account of what we ought to do. However, recognition of one duty leads us to recognition of another, and so we can begin to adjust and complete the picture of what we ought to do on the whole. This is the mutual restriction characteristic of 'wide' duties, or duties of virtue, in general. The only way to find the right balance of practical love and respect, as well as between duties to self and others, is to continually engage with our duties and consider them in context with each other, and with the facts of the particular situation. For this reason, Kant also adds what he calls 'casuistical questions' to some of his discussions of duties of virtue (MM 6:423.17–424.08; MM 6:426.01–32; MM 6:428.01–26; MM 6:431.16–34; MM 6:433.06–434.19; MM 6:437.03–26; MM 6:454.01–28; MM 6:458.01–19). To pick an example concerning the duty to self not to commit suicide and the duty of beneficence to others:

> A man already sensed hydrophobia, effected by the bite of a mad dog; and, after declaring he had never heard of someone who was cured, he took his own life, lest—as he said in a piece of writing he left behind—he also make others unhappy in his doglike madness (the onset of which he already felt). The question is whether he did wrong in this. (MM 6:423.32–424.02)

Kant never resolves these examples, and that is exactly the point. His intention is not to test the reader's comprehension of his ethical system, as if it were an algorithm that always yields a definite moral injunction. Rather, Kant wants to encourage his readers to engage in reflections of their own, recognise apparently conflicting duties, and try to find a resolution that best suffices all demands. Ultimately, he trusts that ordinary agents, if they pay proper attention and reflect thoroughly, will be able to judge what is to be done in the particular situation.

Overall, Kant's central demand when it comes to our treatment of other human beings is that we should treat them with the right balance of practical love and practical respect. We ought to be beneficent to each other while not encroaching upon their affairs too much. When human beings mutually treat each other in this way, Kant calls their relation "friendship" (MM 6:469.17–18). As far as interpersonal morality is concerned, this is his moral ideal.

2.5   KANT'S LIST OF DUTIES TOWARDS OTHERS

Having gained an impression of the architecture of Kant's taxonomy, let us consider the specific duties it contains. Since ethical duties are 'wide' and hence must always be considered in context (with facts and our other duties), it can be somewhat misleading to list them one by one. Kant is well aware of this. His intent is decidedly *not* to present iron laws that must be followed irrespective of the situation. What Kant *does* provide in the *Doctrine of Virtue* is a series of spotlights, emphasising duties which he deems mentionable and in need of explanation.[20] This series should not be understood as an exhaustive list of all a human being's duties. First of all, Kant only lists duties *all* human beings have, independently of our contingent "condition" (MM 6:468.15–16), such as being morally pure or corrupted, educated or uneducated, healthy or sick. Secondly, some all-too-obvious examples of duties and vices do not make Kant's list, such as the prohibition of murder and bodily harm (Sensen 2013, 357). To be sure, such actions also belong in the *Doctrine of Right* (as Sensen points out, ibid.). However, it would seem perfectly in line with the idea of another's happiness as an obligatory end to say that we should *adopt the end of not harming others* in the first place, which would be a duty of virtue.[21] But it is not a duty Kant considers to be in need of particular elucidation.[22]

---

[20] Admittedly, Kant does not frame his own account quite so liberally. For instance, he provides a "division of duties of love" (MM 6:452.10), asserting "They are: A) duties of *beneficence*, B) of *gratitude*, C) of *sympathetic participation*" (MM 6:452.11–12). This suggests that Kant intends his taxonomy to be an exhaustive list. However, first, there seems to be no reason why it would be exhaustive and clear reasons why it is not (too many obvious duties are missing). So it seems more charitable to take Kant to be providing emphases rather than an exhaustive list. Secondly, we can read Kant's "division" quite trivially as a division *of the duties he is about to discuss*, not of all duties there are.

[21] One might object that an end 'not to harm others' is not a positive end, since adopting it consists merely in *not* adopting an end of harming others. This would be a negative duty, not a duty of virtue to adopt a certain end. But there is a difference between merely *not* adopting an end of harming others, and adopting an end *not* to harm others. One can take specific actions in order to avoid harming others, and these are much more specific than simply actions one might take for the sake of ends other than harming others.

[22] Sensen argues that any duty of respect can be made out to be a variant of the prohibition of arrogance, backbiting, and derision (Schönecker 2013, 358f.). A prohibition of the intent to murder a human being would only be an "outward manifestation" of arrogance (Schönecker 2013, 359; see MM 6:463.06). I do not adopt this reading for two reasons: First, it waters down the specificity of Kant's examples. Secondly, it effectively does require

Table 2.2 Kant's list of duties towards others

	Love	*Respect*
Duties of virtue	Beneficence (MM 6:452)	Modesty (MM 6:462)
	Gratitude (MM 6:454)	Respect for others (MM 6:462)
	Sympathetic participation (MM 6:456)	
Vices	Envy (MM 6:458)	Contempt (MM 6:463)
	Ingratitude (MM 6:459)	Arrogance (MM 6:465)
	Malicious glee (MM 6:459)	Backbiting (MM 6:466)
		Derision (MM 6:467)

Kant chooses to focus on a handful of duties of virtue, often paying even more attention to the *vices* opposed to the respective duties. In particular, Kant discusses the following duties and vices[23] (Table 2.2):

At first sight, the listed duties appear like prescriptions of general dispositions that will be conducive to the promotion of happiness overall. And indeed, Kant does explain some of these duties in terms of "propensities" (MM 6:458.28), that is to say, in terms of dispositions. Still, Kant's goal is not simply to provide rules that, on the whole, lead to the promotion of happiness. His point is not that of a rule-utilitarian. Kant's point is rather that for beings like us, promoting the happiness of others requires that we take certain practical-emotional stances and avoid others. These stances are a matter of how we *see* and *set out to treat* others. They are not merely instrumentally conducive to fulfilment of our duty to promote happiness. They are necessary aspects of duty fulfilment, at least for beings like us.

2.6   KANT'S RESTORATIVE PROJECT IN MORAL PHILOSOPHY

Having introduced Kant's conception of moral concern for others, let me add a thought on the *purpose* of this conception. Why, in the first place, does Kant establish the obligatory ends of another's happiness and our

that we read Kant's explicit list as non-exhaustive. *Literal* arrogance, backbiting, and derision are only part of what Kant means to condemn, even on Sensen's reading. So a more liberal reading has little advantage over a literal reading which simply takes Kant's list as non-exhaustive.

[23] Here I list only the duties Kant himself mainly emphasises. In discussing these duties and vices, he however also mentions some further duties, such as placability (MM 6:461.02–03) and alerting friends to their mistakes (MM 6:470.23).

own perfection, his account of love and respect, and his list of duties? This question is worth asking because Kant's project in moral philosophy differs crucially both from that of many neo-Kantian philosophers and that of most animal ethicists today.

On the one hand, Kant's project at this point is *not* to disprove radical moral scepticism or nihilism. This is the aim of many neo-Kantian constructivists who argue that even a moral sceptic or nihilist is implicitly committed to the rational standards from which morality arises (most notably Korsgaard 1986, 1996, and Velleman 2009). To be certain, Kant does consider the possibility that morality might be a "chimera" (G 4:445.08; G 4:407.17) and that the concept of duty might be "empty" (G 4:421.12). His elaborations on morality and freedom in *Groundwork* III and the second *Critique* are intended to tackle this problem to some extent. However, it is not a problem Kant is too concerned with overall. As Timmermann points out, "Kant's problem is the worry of someone who is well disposed towards morality but cannot understand it" (Timmermann 2007a, xxiii). In contrast to a moral sceptic or nihilist, such a person shares at least an *awareness* of her duties, even though she might second-guess herself about whether these duties truly obtain. Accordingly, Kant's central project in moral philosophy is not to disprove an imaginary opponent who is fundamentally opposed to notions of morality and duty. It is rather to use philosophical means to strengthen respect for the moral law, and trust in the concept of duty, for those who are already broadly on board. In the *Groundwork*, he does this by giving the moral law a tangible representation in the various formulas of the Categorical Imperative. The *Doctrine of Virtue*, where we find Kant's substantive account of moral concern, is a continuation of this project. Here, he begins from the moral law and derives from it various duties we already take ourselves to have (see Trampota 2013, 145f.). Thus, Kant means to solidify our trust in our ordinary moral feelings by showing that these feelings have a rational basis. Moral philosophy serves as a reminder that we really do have the duties we typically think we have and that they take logical normative priority over the demands of our inclinations.

On the other hand, in contrast to many animal ethicists today, Kant's primary goal is *not* to establish a philosophical ground for moral objections against widespread moral beliefs and practices. His thought is not meant to be at odds with everyday moral thinking, neither in its terms nor in its upshots (Timmermann 2007a, xii). According to Kant, all human beings have access to the moral law and are basically capable of judging what conforms with it. They are in no desperate need of philosophers to open their eyes to a moral truth that would otherwise be inaccessible. Such a conception would in fact run counter to Kant's aim of instilling trust in ordinary moral feelings.

At first sight, this might come as a disappointment to animal ethicists—at least to those of us who value philosophy's potential to challenge established orders and help people to think differently. An important purpose of contemporary animal ethics is to critique wrongs committed, accepted, and endorsed by an overwhelming majority of human beings. This is possible only if moral philosophy can set people right about their duties. A purely vindicatory project would be doomed to moral standstill.

However, Kant does provide ample grounds for moral criticism. He is far from claiming that most people are morally good, to the contrary (Timmermann 2007a, xvi). Although human beings are at any time *capable* of morality (Timmermann 2007a, xii), we at the same time stand under the influence of inclinations—"a powerful counterweight to all the commands of duty" (G 4:405.05–06). For this reason, the paradigmatic case of a Kantian moral challenge is that duty demands one thing, inclination another, and we are aware of the tension. Usually, we end up acting on inclinations, thus failing to be good. The task of the moral philosopher is to "uphold the strictness and purity of moral principles" (Timmermann 2007b, 182). This is the characteristic way in which a Kantian philosopher criticises bad actions: not by claiming insight into a moral truth hidden to others, but by pointing out that the actions at issue are based on inclination instead of autonomy.

What is more, Kant is well aware that our inclinations lead us to *rationalise* our moral beliefs. In his words, "there arises a *natural dialectic*, that is, a propensity to rationalise against those strict laws of duty and to cast doubt upon their validity, or at least upon their purity and strictness, and, where possible, to make them better suited to our wishes and inclinations" (G 4:405.13–16). So although human beings do not need moral philosophy in order to be capable of acting morally, Kant thinks that moral philosophy can help to *restore* the common moral standpoint in the face of inclination-based rationalisations. Its function is to "clarify, systematize, and vindicate" (Sticker 2017, 85) the thinking of ordinary moral agents and at times to counteract the influence of rationalisations by reminding human beings about the true content and strictness of their duties (Sticker 2017). This is how Kant's approach to moral philosophy enables criticism not just of bad actions, but also of wrongheaded moral beliefs.

It is due to the above conception that Kant's moral philosophy is not just *able* to criticise majority practices and beliefs, but is in fact particularly *strict* in its criticism. There is no such thing as non-culpable moral ignorance in Kant's picture (Timmermann 2007a, xii). If human beings were sincere and attentive enough, in Kant's view, they could always grasp the proper demands of duty, and at heart they would always be able to fulfil these demands. In this way, Kant refuses to let moral agents off the hook, particularly if their wrongs result from a lack of moral reflection.

The idea that certain moral beliefs are convenient human rationalisations should again be familiar to animal ethicists. There is evidence, for instance, that eating meat tends to reduce people's readiness to judge that animals are morally considerable in their own right (Loughnan et al. 2010). As Nussbaum points out, "[animal ethics] is an area in which we will ultimately need good theories to winnow our judgments because our judgments are so flawed and shot through with self-serving inconsistency" (Nussbaum 2001, 1548). Hence, considering how strongly our inclinations favour dismissive moral beliefs about animals, Kant's restorative conception of moral philosophy should seem promising to animal ethicists, particularly to those who are critical of deeply entrenched and rarely questioned exploitation.

While Kant himself develops his taxonomy of ethical duties in the *Doctrine of Virtue* in the context of a restorative project, the resulting system can serve other purposes as well. Most importantly, from the perspective of a contemporary field of 'applied' ethics, Kant's system offers its own ethical vocabulary. Its concepts and distinctions can be used by ethicists to Kantian or non-Kantian ends, provided the vocabulary is at least broadly applicable to their domain of ethics. Kant's taxonomy of ethical duties also doubles as a body of systematic arguments for first-order normative claims—arguments which are often novel and interesting. Consider, for example, Kant's argument that lying is "the greatest violation of a human being's duty to himself" (MM 6:429.04), which suggests that lying wrongs the liar, not just the lie's recipient. The argument gains intricacy the more we consider its relation to Kant's views on lying more broadly, and to his views on morality in general, at the level we would now call metaethical. Such cross-relations give a contemporary ethicist yet more to work with. The same is true, to some extent, for any of Kant's arguments for a first-order normative claim. In this way, Kant's moral philosophy, and the *Doctrine of Virtue* in particular, has great creative potential for philosophers reflecting on our moral relations to others and ourselves.

The main upshot here is that a Kantian framework, if we can get it to include animals in moral concern, will be geared towards a different purpose than standard approaches to animal ethics. Rather than trying to convince the denier of animal moral status or of morality itself, Kantianism for Animals will address itself primarily to those who already share an awareness of duties towards animals and will aim to account for those duties on the basis of an autonomously imposed moral law. Doing so helps to strengthen our commitment to the moral law and to reinforce our trust in ordinary moral feelings of obligation towards animals. It can do so even in opposition to majority practices and beliefs, if they are inclination-driven rationalisations, as many dismissive moral views about animals plausibly are. The resulting system will also double as a body of concepts, distinctions, and arguments that can help contemporary ethicists reflect on our moral relations to others and ourselves.

To sum up this chapter, I have given an account of how Kant conceives of moral concern, placing an emphasis on the ethical duties Kant takes us to have towards each other. Kantian moral concern is a dynamic and complex affair. Duties of different types must be considered in context and brought together by moral judgement. This includes perfect and imperfect duties, duties towards self and others, duties of right and virtue, and duties of love and respect. As far as our treatment of other human beings is concerned, we ought to opt for the right balance between practical love and respect, thus benefitting others without encroaching upon their lives too much. Kant's taxonomy of duties is a helpful and interesting conceptual grid because it forces us to look at our duties from different angles. Attached to it is a philosophical account of moral normativity based on the idea of an autonomously imposed moral law. With the help of this account, we can trace our ordinary moral outlook back to its rational basis, vindicating and refining our ordinary feelings of moral obligation. Whether as a philosophical starting point or as a philosophical interlocutor, Kant's ethical system is an interesting resource to work with. However, Kant gives a radically different treatment to animals than to human beings. In the next chapter, let me explain how animals fit into Kant's ethical system as it stands and why his 'indirect duty approach' to animal ethics is unsatisfactory.

References

Altman, Matthew C. 2011. *Kant and applied ethics: The uses and limits of Kant's practical philosophy.* Malden, MA: Wiley-Blackwell.

Cohen, Carl. 2001. In defense of the use of animals. In *The animal rights debate,* ed. Tom Regan, 29–46. Lanham, MD: Rowman & Littlefield.

DeGrazia, David. 1996. *Taking animals seriously: Mental life and moral status.* Cambridge: Cambridge University Press.

Dombrowski, Daniel A. 1997. *Babies and beasts: The argument from marginal cases.* Champaign, IL: University of Illinois Press.

Fahmy, Meilssa S. 2013. Understanding Kant's duty of respect as a duty of virtue. *Journal of Moral Philosophy* 10: 723–740.

Forkl, Markus. 2001. *Kants System der Tugendpflichten: Eine Begleitschrift zu den Metaphysischen Anfangsgründen der Tugendlehre.* Lausanne: Peter Lang.

Freiin von Villiez, Carola. 2015. Pflichten, vollkommene/unvollkommene. In *Kant-Lexikon,* ed. Marcus Willaschek, Jürgen Stolzenberg, Georg Mohr, and Stefano Bacin, 1757. Berlin: De Gruyter.

Frey, R. G. 1977. Animal rights. *Analysis* 37: 186–189.

Frey, R. G. 1988. Moral standing, the value of lives, and speciesism. *Between the Species: A Journal of Ethics* 4: 191–201.

Garcia, Ernesto V. 2012. A new look at Kantian respect for persons. *Kant Yearbook* 4: 69–89.

Garthoff, Jon. 2020. Against the construction of animal ethical standing. In *Kant and animals,* ed. John J. Callanan and Lucy Allais, 191–212. Oxford: Oxford University Press.

Goodpaster, Kenneth E. 1978. On being morally considerable. *The Journal of Philosophy* 75: 308–325.

Gregor, Mary J. 1963. *Laws of freedom: A study of Kant's method of applying the Categorical Imperative in the "Metaphysik der Sitten".* Oxford: Basil Blackwell.

Gregor, Mary J., ed. 1996. *Immanuel Kant: Practical philosophy.* Translated by Mary J. Gregor. Cambridge: Cambridge University Press.

Hay, Carol. 2013. *Kantianism, liberalism, and feminism: Resisting oppression.* New York: Palgrave Macmillan.

Hayward, Tim. 1994. Kant and the moral considerability of non-rational beings. *Royal Institute of Philosophy Supplement* 36: 129–142.

Herman, Barbara. 2018. We are not alone: A place for animals in Kant's ethics. In *Kant on persons and agency,* ed. Eric Watkins, 174–191. Cambridge: Cambridge University Press.

Hoff, Christina. 1983. Kant's invidious humanism. *Environmental Ethics* 5: 63–70.

Horta, Oscar. 2014. The scope of the argument from species overlap. *Journal of Applied Philosophy* 31: 142–154.

Jaworska, Agnieszka, and Julie Tannenbaum. 2018. The grounds of moral status. Edited by Edward N. Zalta. *The Stanford Encyclopedia of Philosophy.*

Kain, Patrick. 2009. Kant's defense of human moral status. *Journal of the History of Philosophy* 47: 59–101.

Kang, Ji-Young. 2015. *Die allgemeine Glückseligkeit: Zur systematischen Stellung und Funktionen der Glückseligkeit bei Kant.* Berlin: De Gruyter.

Klimchuk, Dennis. 2003. Three accounts of respect for persons in Kant's ethics. *Kantian Review* 8: 38–61.

Korsgaard, Christine M. 1986. Skepticism about practical reason. *The Journal of Philosophy* 83: 5–25.

Korsgaard, Christine M. 1996. *The sources of normativity.* Cambridge: Cambridge University Press.

Korsgaard, Christine M. 2018. *Fellow creatures: Our obligations to the other animals.* Oxford: Oxford University Press.

Loughnan, Steve, Nick Haslam, and Brock Bastian. 2010. The role of meat consumption in the denial of moral status and mind to meat animals. *Appetite* 55: 156–159.

Moran, Kate. 2016. Much obliged: Kantian gratitude reconsidered. *Archiv für Geschichte der Philosophie* 98: 330–363.

Moran, Kate. 2017. Demandingness, indebtedness, and charity: Kant on imperfect duties to others. In *The Palgrave Kant handbook*, ed. Matthew C. Altman, 307–329. London: Palgrave Macmillan.

Nussbaum, Martha C. 2001. Animal rights: The need for a theoretical basis. *Harvard Law Review* 114: 1506–1549.

Pluhar, Evelyn B. 1995. *Beyond prejudice: The moral significance of human and nonhuman animals.* Durham/London: Duke University Press.

Rawls, John. 2000. *Lectures on the history of moral philosophy.* Edited by Barbara Herman. Cambridge, MA: Harvard University Press.

Reath, Andrews. 2013. Formal approaches to Kant's formula of humanity. In *Kant on practical justification*, ed. Mark Timmons and Sorin Baiasu, 201–228. Oxford: Oxford University Press.

Regan, Tom. 2004. *The case for animal rights.* Berkeley/Los Angeles: University of California Press.

Rinne, Pärttyli. 2018. *Kant on love.* Berlin: De Gruyter.

Rowlands, Mark. 2012. *Can animals be moral?* Oxford: Oxford University Press.

Rühl, Ulli F. H. 2015. Pflicht. In *Kant-Lexikon*, ed. Marcus Willaschek, Jürgen Stolzenberg, Georg Mohr, and Stefan Bacin, 1750–1755. Berlin: De Gruyter.

Rutledge-Prior, Serrin. 2019. Moral responsiveness and nonhuman animals: A challenge to Kantian morality. *Ethics and the Environment* 24: 45–76.

Sachs, Benjamin. 2011. The status of moral status. *Pacific Philosophical Quarterly* 92: 87–104.

Schönecker, Dieter. 2013. Duties to others from love (TL 6:448–461). In *Kant's "Tugendlehre": A comprehensive commentary*, ed. Andreas Trampota, Oliver Sensen, and Jens Timmermann, 309–341. Berlin: De Gruyter.

Sensen, Oliver. 2013. Duties to others from respect (TL 6:462–496). In *Kant's "Tugendlehre": A comprehensive commentary*, ed. Andreas Trampota, Oliver Sensen, and Jens Timmermann, 343–363. Berlin: De Gruyter.

Sticker, Martin. 2017. Kant's criticism of common moral rational cognition. *European Journal of Philosophy* 25: 85–108.

Svoboda, Toby. 2012. Duties regarding nature: A Kantian approach to environmental ethics. *Kant Yearbook* 4: 143–163.

Svoboda, Toby. 2014. A reconsideration of indirect duties regarding non-human organisms. *Ethical Theory and Moral Practice* 17: 311–323.

Timmermann, Jens. 2006. Good but not required? Assessing the demands of Kantian ethics. *Journal of Moral Philosophy* 2: 9–27.

Timmermann, Jens. 2007a. *Kant's Groundwork of the Metaphysics of Morals: A commentary*. Cambridge: Cambridge University Press.

Timmermann, Jens. 2007b. Simplicity and authority: Reflections on theory and practice in Kant's moral philosophy. *Journal of Moral Philosophy* 4: 167–182.

Gregor, Mary J., Timmermann, Jens, and Jeanine Grenberg, ed. forthcoming. *Immanuel Kant: The Doctrine of Virtue*. Translated by Mary J. Gregor, Jens Timmermann, and Jeanine Grenberg. Cambridge: Cambridge University Press.

Trampota, Andreas. 2013. The concept and necessity of an end in ethics (TL 6:379–389). In *Kant's "Tugendlehre": A comprehensive commentary*, ed. Andreas Trampota, Oliver Sensen, and Jens Timmermann, 139–157. Berlin: De Gruyter.

Velleman, J. David. 2009. *How we get along*. Cambridge: Cambridge University Press.

Vogt, Katja M. 2009. Duties to others: Demands and limits. In *Kant's ethics of virtue*, ed. Monika Betzler, 219–244. Berlin: De Gruyter.

Warren, Mary A. 1997. *Moral status: Obligations to persons and other living things*. Oxford: Clarendon Press.

Wood, Allen W. 1998. Humanity as an end in itself. In *Kant's Groundwork of the Metaphysics of Morals: Critical essays*, ed. Paul Guyer, 165–188. Lanham, MD: Rowman & Littlefield.

Wood, Allen W. 2007. *Kantian ethics*. Cambridge: Cambridge University Press.

Zöller, Günter. 2013. Idee und Notwendigkeit einer Metaphysik der Sitten (MM 6:205–209, 214–218 und TL 6:375–378). In *Kant's "Tugendlehre": A comprehensive commentary*, ed. Andreas Trampota, Oliver Sensen, and Jens Timmermann, 11–24. Berlin: De Gruyter.

CHAPTER 3

The Case Against Kant's 'Indirect Duty' Approach

3.1   KANT'S 'INDIRECT' ACCOUNT OF DUTIES REGARDING ANIMALS

The basic view Kant endorses on our moral relations to animals is that we do not have any duties towards them (MM 6:442.08–11). At best, we have duties 'regarding' animals (MM 6:443.23–25)—that is, duties that pertain to how we should treat animals. But these are not duties towards the animals themselves. This denial of moral status to animals has made Kant uniquely unpopular among animal ethicists. In response to objections from animal ethicists, Kantians' main line of argument has been that Kant's views are not as repugnant as they—admittedly—sound at first. They point out that Kant recognises an indirect duty to cultivate our capacity for sympathy (MM 6:443.10–16). So we should treat animals with sympathy, even though this is not a duty towards the animals. Enthusiastic readers go so far as to claim that "Kant's protection of animals is quite strong" (Sensen 2011, 134), that his views have "strong implications for our treatment of animals" (Denis 2000, 406), or even that "Kant endorses many of the most important policies of animal rights and animal welfare philosophies" (Altman 2011, 31). Have animal ethicists just failed to understand that a duty of sympathy cultivation is an adequate replacement for moral status?

The answer, I argue in this chapter, is no. Even on a charitable reading, Kant's view on animal ethics suffers from severe shortcomings—severe

N. D. Müller, *Kantianism for Animals*, The Palgrave Macmillan Animal Ethics Series, https://doi.org/10.1007/978-3-031-01930-2_3

enough for us to start looking into developing a Kantian alternative. For animal ethicists, this chapter can double as a critical overview of the debate about Kant's animal ethic and an explanation why they should be interested in new Kantian proposals. Hence, even though this chapter will present objections against a certain part of Kant's philosophy, its intent is altogether constructive. The goal is to further motivate the creation of an alternative Kantian animal ethic that succeeds where Kant's fails. This paves the way for the main discussion of Kantianism for Animals in Part II.

My argument will take the following steps: In the present section, I will briefly recap the main features of Kant's account of animal ethics. Following this recap, I will discuss the two major lines of objection against Kant which have repeatedly appeared in the literature. The first is that there is something awry with the structure of Kant's account (Sect. 3.2). The second is that Kant's view simply demands too little (Sect. 3.3). Though the way in which these traditional objections have been presented in the literature is often a bit rough and ready, I will argue that there is something true in each of them. Before concluding, I will add a third and less traditional line of objection: Kant's view of animal ethics is *not helpful in the way it is supposed to be* (Sect. 3.4). Kantian moral philosophy is meant to reinforce trust in ordinary moral feelings, but Kant has us second-guessing the ordinary feelings of obligation towards animals that he acknowledges we have. Overall, the upshot of this chapter is that Kant's view faces powerful objections that should move us to consider how we can develop an alternative.

Let me begin with the basics: Kant's central view in animal ethics, as stated in §§16–17 of the *Doctrine of Virtue* (MM 6:442.03–443.25.) and the *Collins* lecture notes (*Collins* 27:458–460; *Collins* 27:413), is that there are no duties *towards animals*, but that there is a duty *towards self* to cultivate sympathy and gratitude in our interactions with animals. In the *Doctrine of Virtue*, Kant places his reflections in an "Episodic Section" (MM 6:442.03) towards the end of his discussion of our duties towards self.

The main topic of the "Episodic Section" is the "amphiboly in moral concepts of reflection, to take what is a human being's duty to himself for a duty to others" (MM 6:442.04–06). By an 'amphiboly', Kant means a confusion about the form of our duty, but not about its content. We are right to think that we have a duty *to set the end of treating animals with sympathy and gratitude* (the duty's content), but we are mistaken about the beings *towards whom* we have this duty (the duty's form). Presumably, an 'amphiboly' is not just a momentary confusion we can shake off as soon as we become aware of it. Rather, an 'amphiboly' is a confusion stable upon reflection. Our duty to cultivate sympathy does not cease to *appear* to us like a duty towards others, even after we are made aware that it can only be a duty towards self.[1]

The idea is old—almost as old as the European philosophical tradition itself—that our duty to treat animals with sympathy is not a duty towards the animal, but towards human beings or God. Views to this effect were put forward by Thomas Aquinas, Maimonides, Clement of Alexandria, the Stoics, and according to Plutarch, even by Pythagoras (Sorabji 1993, 129, 173). There is nothing at all original about Kant's view in this regard.

Kant however makes two amendments to the old idea: First, that the duty to treat animals with sympathy is directed towards *self* and not towards *other* human beings or God. We have a duty towards ourselves to cultivate our capacity for sympathy and not harm it, because sympathy for others can make it easier for us to fulfil our duties towards them (MM 6:443.14–15). Recall from Chap. 2 that our duties to self demand that we promote our own moral perfection (MM 6:385.32; MM 6:386.18–387.23; see Sect. 2.4). An important part of this is that we keep ourselves in good moral shape, that we do our best to remain capable of observing our duties. Thus, even though others benefit from our sympathy, our duty to *cultivate* the capacity for sympathy is a duty to self.

It is worth mentioning that Kant's argument for sympathy cultivation therefore does *not* hinge on the empirical claim that cruelty to animals leads to cruelty to human beings, contrary to the standard portrayal of Kant's view among animal ethicists.[2] First of all, *all kinds* of duty-violations

---

[1] Broadie and Pybus understand the term 'amphiboly' more technically as a *transcendental amphiboly*, a notion which Kant discusses in the first *Critique* (CPR B326, Broadie and Pybus 1974, 379). A transcendental amphiboly is a confusion between an object of pure understanding and appearances (ibid.). But Kant does not apply the predicate 'transcendental' to the amphiboly in moral concepts of reflection, nor does he explain it to be a confusion between objects of pure understanding and appearances in the *Doctrine of Virtue*. Hence, Broadie and Pybus's reading seems overspecific. More straightforwardly, we can understand the term 'amphiboly' in general to refer to a confusion between different things which is stable upon reflection. The transcendental amphiboly and the amphiboly in moral concepts of reflection are species of this genus.

[2] The view that Kant's position revolves around this empirical claim is standard in animal ethics. It can be found, for example, in Frey (1987, 50), Rachels (1990, 209), Singer (2002, 244), Kemmerer (2006, 126), Steiner (2011, 89), Rollin (2011, 77), and Aaltola (2012,

against other human beings, not just cruelty, can result if we fail to culti-vate one of morality's motivational aides. For instance, a lack of sympathy might make us more egotistical, more miserly, or more arrogant. More importantly, however, Kant is not so much concerned with the *actual* consequences of sympathy cultivation. We always ought to keep ourselves in good moral condition no matter what, in keeping with the obligatory end of our own moral perfection (Kain 2018, 226). So our duty of sym-pathy cultivation obtains no matter whether we will ever *actually* need to rely on sympathy to observe our duties towards others.

Secondly, Kant adds to the old idea the notion of an 'amphiboly' between duties of different types—the idea that our duties to self decep-tively *appear* like duties towards animals. This helps bring together the denial of duties towards animals with the perspective of ordinary moral agents who do take themselves to have such duties. Whereas Aquinas and others would simply have to contradict these agents' moral experience, Kant at least tries to explain that experience (though he still cannot account for it on its own terms).

Kant's account is the most prominent example of what animal ethicists, following Regan, call an 'indirect duty view' (Regan 2004, 174). In fact, Kant himself asserts that the duty to cultivate sympathy is an 'indirect' duty (MM 6:457.26). He also asserts that it 'belongs indirectly' to our duties, though 'viewed directly' it is a duty towards a human being (MM 6:443.23–25). One should mind, however, that the label 'indirect' has a different meaning in contemporary animal ethics than in Kant's writings. To ward off confusion, let me separate the two meanings. Following Regan (Regan 2004, 150), the standard understanding in animal ethics is the following:

Indirect duty (Regan)

An indirect duty is a duty owed to someone else than its main beneficiary.

For example, imagine a babysitter who has promised to a parent to look after their child for the evening. The duty to make good on this promise is owed to the parent, though its straightforward beneficiary is the child.

---

70). To be fair, the *Collins* lecture notes do report Kant as *asserting* this claim (*Collins* 27:459). But on a charitable reading, Kant's view does not crucially *rely* on this claim. That Kant's views are not so dependent on contingent empirical claims is pointed out by Ripstein and Tenenbaum (2020, 152ff.).

Kant's duty to cultivate sympathy and gratitude towards animals is 'indirect' in this sense.[3] This seems to be what Kant expresses when he uses 'directly' and 'indirectly' as adverbs ('belongs indirectly', 'viewed directly', MM 6:443.23–25). But it is not what he usually means when he uses the label as an adjective. His main use could rather be summarised as follows:

Indirect duty (Kant)

An indirect duty is an action or end which is not itself a duty, but which is an accidental means for fulfilling a duty.

Hence, in contrast to the vocabulary in today's animal ethics, Kantian 'indirect duties' are not truly duties, but merely accidental means we ought to use to fulfil our duties (see Timmermann 2005, 140).[4] For example, consider Kant's duty to promote one's own happiness. There is no such duty in general, Kant insists (MM 6:388.26–28). But there is an 'indirect' duty to promote one's own happiness, insofar as it is a contingent fact that being too unhappy will make it impossible for us human beings to observe our duties (G 4:399.03–07; MM 6:388.17–30). So even though there is no 'direct', or true, duty to promote one's own happiness, there is an 'indirect' duty to secure a certain minimum of happiness that is necessary for autonomy.

Cultivating sympathy and gratitude is an 'indirect' duty in this Kantian sense too, since it is a means for being practically benevolent. Indeed, one could even call Kant's duty *doubly* indirect, since the purpose of *cultivating* sympathy is to be able to *act* on sympathy. But acting on sympathy is

---

[3] Again, Kant would not use the phrase 'owed to' as liberally as Regan—for him, not every duty is owed (MM 6:448.13–14). Still, if we think of the duty to cultivate sympathy as a duty *directed towards* someone else than the main beneficiary (the animal), it is clearly an 'indirect' duty in Regan's sense.

[4] In the lecture notes taken by Kant's student Collins, there is an instance where 'indirect' duty is used in the sense of a duty directed towards someone other than its beneficiary (*Collins* 27:459). However, these lecture notes also contain other inconsistencies with Kant's stated views, such as the claim that all our duties regarding animals are duties towards "other people" (*Collins* 27:413). Kant's stated view is clearly that some of our duties regarding animals are duties towards *self*, not *other people* (MM 6:442.04–06). So we should be aware that the *Collins* notes can contain certain technical errors, and the un-Kantian use of the term 'indirect duty' should not confuse us.

itself only an indirect duty, as Kant points out (MM 6:456.20–27).[5] For beings like us, acting on sympathy is a means to the end of promoting the happiness of others, and this, finally, is a direct duty.

What does Kant's account say we should do? As we have already seen, it is not all about *sympathy*. Kant also gives a prominent place to *gratitude* (MM 6:443.22–24; *Collins* 27:459).[6] We can read Kant more generally as asking us to cultivate any and all of our natural capacities insofar as they are serviceable to morality. Besides sympathy and gratitude, he also mentions the capacity for aesthetic appreciation (MM 6:443.02–09). This is a capacity to value things disinterestedly, which is a prerequisite of morality (MM 6:443.04–08). So we ought to cultivate this capacity in our interactions with our natural environment, be it alive or lifeless (see Chap. 10). However, when it comes to animal ethics, it is sympathy that does the most work for Kant.

Sympathy is taking pleasure in another's joy and displeasure in another's suffering (MM 6:456.20–23). It is an emotional response that takes the feelings of others for its object. While the response matches the valence of others' feelings (positive if positive, negative if negative), it is qualitatively different. For instance, to have sympathy for someone with a toothache is not to *have* a toothache, nor is it to *imagine* having a toothache, nor to feel a pain *similar* to a toothache. It does not require that we put ourselves in their shoes, but only that we feel a certain unpleasant emotional response at the sight of their suffering. This makes it possible for us to sympathise with others whose experiences are qualitatively very unlike ours, so long as we can discern the valence of their feelings. However, sympathy is also clearly distinct from stronger feelings of community such as solidarity (in the sense of recognising a common plight) and from what Gruen (2015) calls 'entangled empathy' (which would be an ongoing cognitive and emotional process of reflecting on one's relations with another).

When it comes to the *cultivation* of sympathy, we can think of it as the preservation and strengthening of two connections: first, the bond between the perception of joy and suffering in others and our own

---

[5] At this point (MM 6:456.24–26), Kant calls the duty to use sympathy for beneficence a "conditional" duty, not an "indirect" one. The "condition" at issue is however our duty of beneficence. This indicates that we must treat acting on sympathy as a contingent means to the end of fulfilling our duty of beneficence, making our use of sympathy an indirect duty.

[6] The idea that we ought to be grateful towards animals, particularly horses and dogs (MM 6:443.22–23), can also be found in Plutarch (Sorabji 1993, 215).

covalent sympathetic feelings; secondly, the bond between our own sympathetic feelings and benevolent action-intentions. Ideally, when we see
someone suffering, we respond *affectively* with sympathy, and then
respond *practically* with an action-intention to help. Of course, this does
not yet ensure that we act in accordance with duty, let alone *from* duty.
But at least, the inclinations of a sympathetic person are generally more in
line with duty, making it easier to act from duty. Sympathy cannot guarantee morality, but it can remove some major obstacles. This is what Kant
asserts when he writes that sympathy is "a natural predisposition that is
very serviceable to morality in one's relations with other people" (MM
6:443.14–15).

Our duty of cultivation admits of a negative and a positive dimension.
In its negative dimension, our duty demands that we *avoid weakening* the
bonds between the perception of suffering, our sympathetic response, and
benevolent action-intentions. As Kant puts it:

> violent and at the same time cruel treatment of animals is far more intimately
> opposed to a human being's duty to himself, because his fellow feeling for
> their suffering is thereby dulled and a natural predisposition that is very
> serviceable to morality in one's relations with other people is thereby weak-
> ened and little by little erased. (MM 6:443.11–16)

Hence, we violate our duty of sympathy cultivation in the most egre-
gious way if we act for the sake of cruelty, that is, if we set out to derive
pleasure from others' suffering. But Kant's account also plausibly prohib-
its *desensitisation*: numbing oneself to the perception of suffering. One
could also emphasise the connection to our benevolent action-intentions:
Kant can plausibly prohibit that we remain *indifferent* in light of our sympathetic responses. Once we respond affectively to the perception of suffering, we must act in accordance with our emotional response so as to
retain it as a resource to aid moral motivation. Besides outright cruelty,
Kant also takes the overworking of animals to be a violation of duty (MM
6:443.17–19), as well as all animal experiments "merely for the sake of
speculation" if other methods are available (MM 6:443.19–21). In sum,
anything we do which weakens the bond between our perception of suffering, covalent sympathetic feelings, and benevolent action-intentions is
against our duty. Sympathy is a morally helpful machine that needs
maintaining.

The positive aspect of cultivation, which Kant also mentions, is that we ought to bring ourselves into situations in which we can indulge in sympathetic feelings and act on them. To use his example, we ought not to avoid poor neighbourhoods, but purposely walk through them, perceive the suffering of the poor, and then act on our sympathetic feelings (MM 6:457.29–35). With regard to animals, however, Kant puts more emphasis on the positive cultivation of *gratitude*, asserting that "gratitude for the long service of an old horse or dog (just as if they were members of the household [*Hausgenossen*]) belongs indirectly to a human being's duty" (MM 6:443.22–24). So we are to indulge in feelings of gratitude and act on them, so as to further increase our capacity for gratitude.

As an aside, although the term '*Hausgenossen*' translates literally to 'members of the household', the term used to refer to the lowest class of farm labourers, who did not own a house, land, or livestock, and who were explicitly excluded from using their communities' common land (Otto 1900, 334). Thus, when Kant likens animals to '*Hausgenossen*', he likens them to what is arguably the most disenfranchised class of human beings in the rural social structure of his day. *Hausgenossen* are labourers who are not considered to belong to the communities they serve and towards whom members of those communities have almost no duties. Nevertheless, of course one can be grateful to a *Hausgenosse* for their service, even though full members of the community do not strictly owe them gratitude for anything. Doing so marks us out as generally good cultivators of our own capacity for gratitude. So Kant's comparison is not quite as heartwarming as it appears at first sight. It merely emphasises once more that our duty to treat animals with gratitude is not a duty *towards*, but only *regarding* them.

As a first upshot, animal ethicists should recognise that there is more to Kant's account of animal ethics than just his denial of duties towards animals. In particular, Kant is far from claiming that we may treat animals in whatever way we please. This point is all the more important for those who take a critical stance towards Kant. If they bank on the initial repugnance of Kant's denial of duties towards animals, Kantians will be right to point to the true intricacies of his view. Unfortunately, much of the debate between animal ethicists and Kantians follows this dialectic. In the coming two sections, let me explain the two main lines of argument that have been advanced against Kant by animal ethicists. In each case, Kantians have defended Kant by expounding his indirect-duty view. However, in each case, I claim that the defence has been overstated. As much as we should read Kant's text charitably, we should acknowledge the true strength of the objections he faces. First, let me begin with structural criticisms: Is there anything *inconsistent* about Kant's view?

3.2   STRUCTURAL PROBLEMS OF KANT'S ACCOUNT

Many animal ethicists share the impression that there must be something structurally wrong with Kant's 'indirect duty' account (e.g. Warren 1997, 51; Cavalieri 2001, 49; Zamir 2007, 28). Some of Kant's readers suppose that his view must be a mere "auxiliary construction" (Wolf 1990, 34; Timmermann 2005, 132). Between the claim that we have no duties towards animals and the claim that treating them badly cultivates an immoral disposition, something just does not seem to fit. But what *exactly* does not fit? The literature offers several distinct answers. In this section, let me distinguish three structural objections and explain why each fails in its stated form. Afterwards, I will add a novel, more robust structural objection against Kant.

The first structural objection takes issue with Kant's supposed view that there is nothing objectionable about animal cruelty 'in itself', but that it still cultivates an objectionable disposition. Call this the *'alright in itself objection'*. One of its earliest instances was put forward by Nozick:

> Some say people should not [kill animals] because such acts brutalize them and make them more likely to take the lives of persons, solely for pleasure. These acts that are morally unobjectionable in themselves, they say, have an undesirable moral spillover. [...] But why should there be such a spillover? If it is, in itself, perfectly all right to do anything at all to animals for any reason whatsoever, then provided a person realizes the clear line between animals and persons and keeps it in mind as he acts, why should killing animals tend to brutalize him and make him more likely to harm or kill persons? (Nozick 1974, 36)

Although Nozick did not explicitly address this objection to Kant, the passage is often understood as a point of criticism against Kant's view (e.g. Franklin 2005, 38; Wolf 2012, 42FN). If Nozick is indeed talking about Kant, he diagnoses him with the following contradiction: On the one hand, Kant thinks that nothing at all is wrong with animal cruelty 'in itself', and on the other, he holds that there is so much wrong with it that its evil threatens to 'spill over' into the human domain.

But Nozick is mistaken.[7] First, as mentioned before in Sect. 3.1 above, it is decidedly *not* the case that Kant sees animal cruelty as merely instrumentally bad—as morally unobjectionable save for its bad consequences for other people. According to Kant's account, we have a duty towards self to cultivate our natural capacities insofar as they are serviceable to morality. Sympathy is one of these capacities, and cruelty damages it. So anytime we act cruelly, we violate a duty towards self, *no matter whether any other human beings ever come to harm from it*. So there is no sense in which Kant claims that animal cruelty is 'alright in itself', to the contrary.

For the same reason, the image of a 'spillover' cannot accurately reflect Kant's view of the evil of animal cruelty. It falsely suggests that Kant is concerned with an escalation of duty-violations of the same kind, as if his only worry was that an animal's tormentor might one day graduate to tormenting human beings. Kant's point is rather that we have a general duty towards self to cultivate our natural capacities insofar as they are serviceable to morality, and by being cruel, we violate this duty. Hence, the inconsistency Nozick points out is not Kant's.[8]

A second type of structural objection takes issue with Kant's claim that moral restrictions apply to our treatment of animals, despite their status as 'things'. Call this the *'ordinary things objection'*. Broadie and Pybus present it as follows:

> [Kant's] argument therefore is that if we use certain things, viz. animals, as means, we will be led to use human beings as means. If this argument were generalized, Kant would have to say that using things as means would lead us to treat rational beings as means. And Kant cannot avoid this generalization of his argument, since he cannot point to a morally relevant characteristic which differentiates animals from other things which, he would say, we can use as means. (Broadie and Pybus 1974, 382f.)

[7] Here I omit the point that Nozick, if he is indeed talking about Kant, suggests that Kant condemns *killing* animals. This is not the case (MM 6:443.16–17). Kant is concerned with *cruelty* and *ingratitude*, not with killing. Evidently, this is not a substantial counter to Nozick, since the 'alright in itself objection' does not rest on any point about killing in particular. So I simply discuss Nozick's point as if he had been talking about cruelty all along.

[8] Here I focus on showing that Kant is not the proper target of Nozick's objection. I might add, however, that Nozick's objection appears to fail on philosophical grounds too. It can be perfectly coherent to say that something is alright in itself, but morally bad because it might escalate into moral evils. If it were the case, say, that watching violent films led to violent behaviour, we could say that watching violent films is alright in itself, but bad due to its 'moral spillover'.

The claim at issue here is that Kant commits himself to this inconsistent set of propositions: We must not use animals as means, and any rule that applies to animals applies to all other ordinary things, and we may use some things as means.

This is not the most robust version of the 'ordinary things objection'. One problem with it is that it ascribes to Kant a patently absurd view, namely that one must never use anything as a means (see Broadie and Pybus 1974, 382). If Kant were committed to this view, inconsistency would be the least of his worries. Another problem was pointed out early on by Regan (1976, 471; 2004, 180): Kant never asserts that we must not *use animals as means*. He is concerned with *cruelty* and *ingratitude*. There is nothing to suggest that Kant believes that using animals as means leads to using persons as means. And even if he did believe this, there is still an important difference between using persons *as means* and using them as *mere* means. So it is not clear that cultivating a disposition to use others as means would even be morally problematic to Kant—this might simply be a disposition to recognise others' potential helpfulness, without denigrating their importance as moral patients.

However, these counter-arguments pick up on idiosyncratic weaknesses of Broadie and Pybus's particular version of the 'ordinary things objection'. Circumventing these weaknesses, we could still say that Kant gets tangled up in an inconsistency by claiming that no special moral rules apply to things, but special moral rules apply to animals, who are things.[9] But this line of objection would be mistaken too, for although Kant does assert that animals are things (G 4:428.20–21; Anth 7:127.08), he never declares them to be *things just like all others* (see Sect. 6.3 below). The point of Kant's 'indirect duty' account is exactly that animals are things of a special sort, insofar as they can experience pleasure and suffering (as Herman also points out, Herman 2018, 177). This makes them the proper object of sympathy. The same cannot be said about unfeeling objects. So the 'ordinary things objection' fails.

A third type of structural objection argues that Kant cannot claim that cruelty damages a moral capacity if there are no duties towards animals

---

[9] This argument is also advanced by Wolf, who poses the rhetorical question why special rules should apply to animals if they are just like rocks and cars (Wolf 1990, 36). This overlooks that Kant acknowledges that animals are capable of feeling pleasure and pain, and thus are appropriate objects of our sympathy, while rocks and cars are not.

which cruelty inherently violates. We could call this the '*no moral damage objection*'. As Zamir puts it:

> the Kantian's appeal to a notion of humanity that one distorts if one is cruel to animals seems to smuggle through the backdoor a tacit recognition that animals can be wronged (rather than merely 'harmed'). Why else should cruel acts make for a flawed humanity if animals are morally neutral entities? (Zamir 2007, 28)

Zamir's idea is that cruelty can only be damaging to our humanity if it is a *moral transgression*. After all, in the Kantian literature 'humanity' should be understood to designate a set of essentially *moral* capacities, including autonomy and the capacity to observe duties. If these moral capacities are to be damaged by cruelty, cruelty must be a type of moral transgression, a violation of some duty. But if there is a duty-violation in any act of cruelty towards animals, there must exist some duty we are violating, and this duty could be directed towards nobody but the animal. So in claiming that animal cruelty harms our humanity, Kant has tacitly assumed that there are duties towards animals.[10]

Contrary to this objection, however, Kant never claims that animal cruelty damages our *humanity*. He does not assert that cruelty damages our autonomy or our capacity to recognise and act from duties. Animal cruelty is damaging to *natural capacities that are serviceable to morality*. It erodes the connection between the perception of joy and suffering, natural sympathetic responses, and benevolent action-intentions. This amounts to damaging a tool in humanity's toolbox, not humanity itself. Hence, nothing in Kant's picture commits him to the claim that there are duties towards animals. The 'no moral damage objection' misses its target.

In summary, previous objections of inconsistency against Kant fail. Of course, this does not show that Kant's account is structurally sound. It merely shows that we must be precise about which inconsistency we mean to diagnose. I want to suggest that Kant has no structural problems at all when it comes to the question whether there *actually exist* any duties towards animals. He answers unambiguously in the negative, and no part of his account commits him to the affirmative. Things get tricky for Kant, however, if we refine the question: Are duties towards non-rational beings strictly *unintelligible* or are they *intelligible but non-existent*? As I will now

---

[10] Wolf also voices this objection (Wolf 2012, 43).

argue, Kant is committed to both at the same time, and this is the true structural problem of his view. Call this the '*intelligibility objection*'.

The problem arises as follows: The starting point for Kant's account of animal ethics is that duties towards animals are unintelligible. Such duties cannot exist, and as Broadie and Pybus are right to point out, "this is a logical 'cannot'" (Broadie and Pybus 1974, 379). The reason why there can be no duties towards animals according to Kant is that *directionality* is a feature of our duties that can only obtain between rational beings (this difficulty will be the topic of Chap. 5). To say that a duty is directed 'towards' someone is already to say that their will necessitates us under a shared moral law (see MM 6:442.10–11). But then, duties can necessarily only obtain towards beings who share the moral law, who must be rational beings. And so, 'duty towards a non-rational being' is a contradiction in terms. This is essentially what Kant asserts when he says that "a human being has duties only to human beings (himself and others), since his duty to any subject is moral constraint by that subject's will" (MM 6:442.08–11).

But now enters Kant's innovative addition to traditional anti-cruelty doctrine, the 'amphiboly': What is truly a duty towards self appears like a duty towards someone else. This allows Kant to endorse that we have no duties towards animals while at the same time acknowledging that we all feel as though we had such duties. The trouble is that in order for any-thing to *appear like* a duty towards a non-rational being, such duties must at the very least be intelligible. By way of analogy, a square can *appear like a trapezoid* when viewed from an angle. But it cannot *appear like a four-sided triangle*. A part of a film set may *appear like a wooden barn* from a distance, but it cannot *appear like a wooden barn made entirely of metal*. And likewise, if we are to *confuse* any of our duties for duties towards a non-rational being, then duties towards non-rational beings must at the very least be intelligible, even if they do not happen to exist. This leaves us with an inconsistent pair of claims: Duties towards animals are unintelli-gible and must be explained away, but in the process of explaining them away as illusions or confusions, we have presupposed that they are intelli-gible. This is the true structural problem of Kant's 'indirect duty' view.

A defender of Kant's account could respond as follows: What is intelli-gible are *duties towards furry, feathery, and scaly creatures*, provided we think of them as rational beings. All that is strictly unintelligible are *duties towards non-rational beings*.[11] But this response forces us to claim that

---

[11] I thank Jens Timmermann for pointing this out.

ordinary moral agents do not just mistake duties to self for duties to others, but that they also mistake non-rational beings for rational beings. This line of reasoning is not attractive. Ordinary moral agents might simply insist that they are *not* thinking of animals as rational beings whenever they feel obligated towards them. I certainly am not. So this counter to the 'intelligibility objection' increases Kant's friction with ordinary moral phenomenology rather than decreasing it.

Another counter-argument to the 'intelligibility objection' could be that Kant never said that our feelings of obligation were always coherent. Something might vaguely appear to us like a duty we have, even though the thought of it turns out to be unintelligible under scrutiny. So we might, incoherently, have the impression that we have something like a duty towards a non-rational being. But this response again forces us to suppose that moral agents fall prey to yet another failing. Not only do they confuse duties of different types, but they fail to have coherent moral feelings altogether. Hence, this response fundamentally undermines trust in ordinary moral feelings rather than solidifying it. It hence runs counter to one of Kant's main aims in moral philosophy (see Sect. 2.6 above). As far as I can see, there simply is no straightforward response that saves Kant from the intelligibility objection.

At the same time, note that the 'intelligibility objection' does not attack the very idea of an 'amphiboly in moral concepts of reflection'. Duties of different kinds can be confused for each other, so long as they are all intelligible. Consider again the duty to cultivate our sympathy. This duty may appear to us like a duty *towards other human beings*, when it is really a duty towards self. No inconsistency arises. It only arises when we try to use the 'amphiboly' to *explain away* feelings of obligation towards beings towards whom, supposedly, there necessarily cannot be any duties.

To avoid the intelligibility objection, we however need to be careful in our use of the 'amphiboly'. We must not use it to explain away feelings of obligation towards beings who do not qualify as finite rational beings—including not just animals, but also plants, lifeless nature, and God. In Kant's view, there necessarily cannot be any duties towards any of these beings (MM 6:442.19–25). He explains away any feelings to the contrary in just the same way as he explains away feelings of obligation towards animals. But is it a big loss if we cannot use the 'amphiboly' to this end? I suggest that it is not. As for plants and lifeless nature, it seems doubtful in the first place whether ordinary agents have strong feelings of obligation 'towards' them. Kant's own example is the obligation we feel not to destroy beautiful plants or delicate crystallisations (MM 6:443.08–09). Do ordinary agents really consider themselves obligated *towards* these things? I do not think I do.

Feelings of obligation towards God pose a more serious challenge, since many people might sincerely insist that they feel obligated directly towards God. However, feelings of faith admit of a different conceptualisation and explanation altogether. If we feel obligated 'towards' God, we likely do not think that God is on the receiving end of a moral relation, that he is a moral patient. We might take ourselves to 'owe' things to God, but not in the way we 'owe' things to other people. What is at issue here is rather the recognition of God as the *authority* of our obligations. God is not on the receiving end of duty. He is the ultimate authority to which the moral agent has to answer. Kant has more than enough resources to account for this recognition of divine authority. Indeed, Kant argues that we should think of all our duties as *divine commands* (MM 6:487.08–25; see also Anth 7:074.03–07; MM 6:152.33–37; MM 6:099:10–13), though certainly not as *duties towards God* (MM 6:486.02–03). And so, feelings of obligation towards God do not need to be explained away by appeal to the 'amphiboly'. Ultimately, feelings of obligation towards *animals* pose the only serious challenge to Kant in ordinary moral phenomenology, and only here does he truly need the 'amphiboly'.

Conversely, the idea of an 'amphiboly' would not have to lose its role in a Kantian framework which accommodates duties towards animals. Once we accept duties towards animals as intelligible, there can again be illusions. The duty to cultivate sympathy would still be a duty to self but may appear like a duty towards animals. But now, the statement of this confusion no longer leads into inconsistency.

To summarise, the *alright in itself objection*, the *ordinary things objection*, and the *no moral damage objection* all fail. But according to the *intelligibility objection*, Kant's 'indirect duty' view suffers from a structural problem after all. So the 'indirect duty' account must go. On the one hand, this leaves Kant without an explanation for ordinary feelings of obligation towards animals, which is a pity. On the other, it gives Kantians an opportunity to rethink the conditions of interpersonal moral obligation. Is it really so important to Kant's ethical system that duties 'towards' a being are thought of as duties arising from interpersonal constraint under a shared moral law? In Chap. 5, I will argue that it is not. Next up, however, let me consider the other main line of objection against Kant's 'indirect duty' account in the literature.

3.3   SUBSTANTIVE SHORTCOMINGS OF KANT'S ACCOUNT

Besides those who object to the structure of Kant's view, there are those who object to its substantive upshots. It simply does not demand enough to be plausible. Schopenhauer objected that according to Kant's account, "one is only to have compassion on animals for the sake of practice, and they are as it were the pathological phantom on which to train one's sympathy with men! [...] I regard such tenets as odious and revolting" (Schopenhauer 1915, 94). In a similar vein, Hoff asserted: "Kant's most serious shortcomings where animals are concerned are not logical but moral" (Hoff 1983, 67). Both Schopenhauer and Hoff react to Kant not just with theoretical disagreement, but with righteous anger. Their wrath is directed less at any particular argument of Kant's, but rather at the moral offence of condoning indifference and exploitation.

Of course, an argument along these lines can succeed only if there is some prior moral standard by which we can condemn indifference and exploitation. For Schopenhauer, this standard comes with his own views he develops in the *Basis of Morality* (Schopenhauer 1915). But then, his criticism of Kant's stance on animals is ultimately a proxy for more fundamental disagreements in moral philosophy. Hoff, on the other hand, makes it explicit that she does not base her ethical theorising on any particular system of moral philosophy, but on ordinary moral intuitions:

> In the absence of good arguments in favor of a dogmatic and exclusive humanism, we may trust our moral intuitions. The well-being of an animal appears to be an intrinsically valuable state of affairs, and attempts to view it otherwise are unconvincing, unsatisfactory, and finally, perverse. (Hoff 1983, 68)

Hoff emphasises the intuition that we ought generally to be concerned with animal well-being, that it is wrong to be indifferent to it. The objection is that Kant's view allows human beings to treat animals with indifference and that it therefore clashes with a widespread moral intuition. Call this the '*indifference objection*'.[12]

---

[12] As a derivative of the indifference objection, Zamir objects that according to Kant's view, human beings become "morally free game" (Zamir 2007, 28) if they lose their autonomy. What I will say about Hoff's objection applies, by extension, to Zamir's: Kant does not license total indifference, even though he still licenses too much of it.

Although the relation of Kant's moral philosophy to 'moral intuitions' is complicated, the standard Kantian move has not been to claim blanket immunity against all appeals to intuition.[13] Rather, the main counter is that it does not matter for a duty's *material*—what the duty prescribes—towards whom it is directed (Hayward 1994, 133; Denis 2000, 418; Herman 2018, 188; Ripstein and Tenenbaum 2020, 147). The same material can be prescribed by a duty to self and by a duty to others. And so long as there is *some* duty to treat animals well, the argument goes, it does not matter towards whom exactly it is directed. To further support the Kantian position, many emphasise the fact that Kant takes duties to self very seriously (Baranzke 2005, 340; Sensen 2011, 134; Svoboda 2012, 161; 2014, 316 f.; Camenzind 2018, 55). Duties to self are neither optional nor weaker than duties towards others. Therefore, defenders argue, Kant makes all the necessary moral demands with all the necessary urgency.

There is something true in this Kantian response: The same end or action can indeed be prescribed either by a duty to self or by a duty to others. But this is not enough to shield Kant from the moral criticism of Schopenhauer and Hoff. For if we flatly deny that there are duties towards certain beings, this denial *does* restrict what our duties 'regarding' these beings can demand. The form and content of our duties are not completely decoupled.

To see the problem more clearly, consider this: If duties can only be directed towards human beings, there can only be duties 'regarding' animals insofar as those animals stand in some relation to human beings. The relevant relation for Kant is that of affecting the natural capacities of human beings insofar as they are serviceable to morality (which I will now call 'natural-moral capacities' for short). But unfortunately, what is good for animals is not always good for our natural-moral capacities. And what is bad for animals is not always bad for our capacities. We can visualise this using Table 3.1.

---

[13] One could argue that transcendental philosophy provides a methodological alternative to intuitions-based theorising. If one then claimed that no such thing as an 'intuition' is ever a legitimate measuring stick for the results of transcendental arguments, one could deflect all intuition-based, substantive moral criticism. However, one would have to be a particularly staunch Kantian in the first place to go along with this line of reasoning. I do not pursue this line of argument further because that is not the audience of this book. To my knowledge, it is also not an argument that anyone in the literature has put forward to defend Kant's 'indirect duty' view.

Table 3.1   What is good for animals versus for our capacities

		For natural-moral capacities		
		Good	Neutral	Bad
For animals	Good	Acting on sympathy, being grateful, appreciating natural beauty		
	Neutral			
	Bad			Acting cruelly, being ungrateful, wantonly destroying natural beauty

The limitation of Kant's view is that he is bound to morally encourage behaviours in the left-hand column, be indifferent about behaviours in the middle column, and discourage behaviours in the right-hand column. This may not be so problematic as long as we focus on the cells in which good matches with good, and bad with bad—that is, the upper-left, middle, and lower-right cells. Acting on sympathy for animals, for instance, is usually good both for animals and for our natural-moral capacities. Acting cruelly, conversely, is bad in both respects. But Kant's view becomes increasingly counterintuitive the more we consider behaviours that belong in the other cells of the table.

It would be convenient if there simply were no such behaviours—if the good of our capacities and the good of animals always aligned. But this is not the case. The most obvious counterexamples are behaviours which belong in the lower-middle cell: behaviours that are neutral to our natural-moral capacities but are clearly bad for animals. Consider that the suffering and death of billions of animals per annum today is not, for the most part, the result of cruelty. It is the result of what Noske called the "animal industrial complex" (Noske 1997, 22): a dynamic legal and economic system of animal use which effectively shields most of its participants from perceiving the suffering that their actions help to inflict. Participation in this system and failure to help dismantle it is bad for animals, but for most consumers, workers, and investors, it is utterly neutral to their moral capacities. Kant's view of the morality of human-animal relations begins only where animal joy and suffering are *perceived*. It has nothing to say about those of us who contribute to animal suffering without perceiving that suffering. Notice that the point here is not about affective or practical *indifference* to suffering of which we are aware—Kant could condemn that. The point is that we never become aware of most of the suffering to which we contribute in the first place. Where there is no perception of suffering, there is no opportunity to cultivate sympathy.

Even if we narrow our view to those on the frontlines of inflicting animal suffering, such as slaughterhouse workers, Kant's view has trouble casting any critical light on what they do. As Carruthers has pointed out, "almost any legitimate, non-trivial motive is sufficient to make [an] action separable from a generally cruel or insensitive disposition" (Carruthers 2002, 159; see also Fischer 2018, 253). Even factory farming and industrial slaughter, arguably the greatest moral atrocities committed against animals in our time, are not *cruel*, strictly speaking (Hsiao 2017). That is, people engage in these practices without *taking any pleasure* in the perception of suffering. We may even suppose that most engage in the professional infliction of animal suffering with a certain *pro tanto* regret. They may very well sympathise with animals but judge that other concerns override their beneficent action-intention in this case (such as earning a living, or providing other people with products they are presumed to need). The worker's regret is evidence that their sympathy is *not* isolated from action. Were they to encounter *human* suffering, or indeed animal suffering outside the context of the animal industrial complex, they *would* still be inclined to help. It is only within a very specific economic context that they judge the intention to help to be insufficient to determine action. Hence, not only is the worker not being cruel, but they are not even desensitising themselves. Kant only has grounds to object once the worker's regret starts to fade. This is a serious restriction of his view.

There are also examples of behaviours that are *good* for our capacities, but *bad* for animals. Suppose we sacrifice a bull to the Hellenic gods (or kill a sheep to serve to a benefactor who is guest of honour), cultivating our capacity for gratitude, for instance. And even if we turn to sympathy, there can be examples where cultivating our capacities is bad for animals. Suppose we mistake an animal's suffering for pleasure due to an anthropomorphic misinterpretation. The facial expression of a hyperventilating cat can resemble an excited human smile. Imagine that I take a cat on a car ride. The cat enters a state of panic, but I keep confusing expressions of panic with expressions of wondrous enthusiasm. In my uninformed state I experience sympathetic pleasure for the cat. And I think to myself that going on more of these car rides together would be a great way to positively cultivate my capacity for sympathy. Kant has no grounds on which to object to me. This is a case in which promoting suffering cultivates sympathetic capacities in a way that is serviceable to our moral relations to human beings, in whom the respective expressions *would in fact be* expressions of joy!

There are also things which would be *good* for animals, but *bad* for our capacities. These things Kant must discourage, counterintuitively. For instance, it would be good for animals if we set out to confront their true suffering at the hands of human beings and then do something about it. But human beings inflict so much violence on so many animals that confronting even just a portion of it threatens to erode our natural-moral capacities. First, because our capacity to sympathise is limited, there is a point at which we develop 'compassion fatigue' (Figley 1995), an inability to sympathise any longer. In this way, confronting animal suffering might very well make us less sympathetic to human beings. So Kant must ask us to look away. Secondly, confronting the full scope of animal suffering may lead to a degree of misanthropy (Wuensch et al. 2002). In fact, it has been explicitly argued in the philosophical literature that misanthropy is a *morally appropriate* response to how people treat animals (Cooper 2018). But Kant emphatically discourages behaviours that lead to misanthropy (MM 6:450.22–29; MM 6:466.18–25) or which might diminish our respect for an individual person (MM 6:472.01–07). So Kant must, once again, discourage us from paying attention to most animal suffering, lest we lose respect for those who inflict it. In this case, what is good for animals is bad for our natural-moral capacities. But if something *can* be done about animal suffering, provided we confront it, it is counterintuitive that we should wilfully ignore it.

The listed behaviours have to do either with ignorance of animal suffering or with indifference to it. Kant's account of animal ethics is all about how our treatment of animals affects our capacities. But what really affects our capacities is a package deal of certain *perceptions* of pleasure and suffering, our sympathetic *responses*, and our *intentions* to help or harm. As soon as one element of this package becomes unlinked, Kant's argument ceases to be relevant. The intentions become unlinked from the package as soon as we harm animals out of innocuous, unrelated motives, as in the case of the sacrificed bull. Perceptions of suffering become unlinked as soon as we miss or misinterpret animal expressions, as in the case of the hyperventilating cat. Sympathetic responses become unlinked as soon as indulging in and acting out of sympathy harms our capacities rather than cultivating them, as in the cases of compassion fatigue and misanthropy.

This is not a comprehensive list of all counterexamples to Kant's view, but rather a template for generating as many new counterexamples as we like. And what such counterexamples bring out is not that Kant's view has little loopholes here and there. They bring out the way in which animals truly do not matter, if they do not matter for their own sake. A degree of moral indifference towards animals—an objectionable degree!—is inevitable if we deny that we have duties towards them. This is, in effect, a refined version of Hoff's 'indifference objection'.

To this line of objection, one might respond with an even stronger reading of Kant's position: If ignorance and indifference are the problem, *attention* is the solution. That is, one could argue that like sympathy, gratitude, and aesthetic appreciation, our capacity to pay close attention to others and their experiences is a natural capacity serviceable to morality. Along similar lines, Denis has suggested that we have an imperfect duty to keep ourselves informed about how our actions impact others (Denis 2000, 416), and Svoboda has argued that "[b]y ignoring the plights of animals whose suffering one could alleviate, [...] one misses a chance to cultivate virtuous dispositions" (Svoboda 2012, 158).

But this line of argument only leads to more trouble. For what could it mean to cultivate our attention for others *insofar as it is serviceable to morality*? Surely, the kind of attention for others we ought to cultivate must help us recognise and observe our duties towards others. In the case of a human being, we ought to pay attention to their suffering and not look away *because we may have a duty to relieve their suffering*. And if we mistake another human being's suffering for joy, we have failed to pay proper attention *because we have a duty to relieve another's actual suffering* (as opposed to the mere appearance of suffering). But in the case of animals, there are no such duties to anchor our moral attention. Hence, there is no reason why cultivating our capacity for moral attention would require that we pay any thorough attention to animals' joy and suffering. It suffices that we react in the right way to what we superficially perceive as their pleasure and suffering, whenever we happen to perceive it.

On the whole, then, we can grant that duties to self give rise to *some* prescriptions about how we ought to treat animals. But they do not give rise to *just any prescriptions we like*. There are severe restrictions to what Kant's 'indirect duty' account can reasonably demand. These restrictions are too severe to survive scrutiny in the light of the moral intuitions that motivated Hoff's (Hoff 1983) substantive criticism of Kant. The restrictions are also too severe to make Kant's view a helpful resource for a critique of the animal industrial complex. Though the point has been overstated in the literature that Kant authorises *total* moral indifference regarding animals, Kant's account does end up condoning *by far too much* indifference towards animals. In a refined version, the indifference objection is sound.

In the face of the indifference objection, one could argue that no matter whether our duties regarding animals demand very much, they at least give great *weight* to what they demand. It has been suggested in the literature that Kant considers *perfect* duties to self to be a particularly important kind of duty and that our duties regarding animals belong in this privileged class (Baranzke 2005, 340; Camenzind 2018, 55; Herman 2018, 188). However, even this well-intentioned attempt at painting Kant's view in a positive light fails: First, there is no reason to think that all our duties regarding animals are of this specific kind. A duty to *positively* cultivate our sympathy, for instance, is straightforwardly imperfect (Svoboda 2012, 154). In general, any duty of any type whatsoever can be a duty 'regarding' animals if animals are affected by it, since that is all the label 'regarding' denotes. Secondly, whether a duty is perfect or imperfect does not indicate how important or stringent it is. Both types of duties have obligatory force, and according to the main text of the *Metaphysics of Morals*, neither allows for inclination-based exceptions (MM 6:390.10–12). So the suggestion is misleading that Kant assigns a "place of honour" to duties regarding animals (as Baranzke puts it, Baranzke 2005, 340). Their place is no more honourable than that of any other duties.

To be sure, Kant does take duties to self seriously. The *Collins* lecture notes even have him asserting that duties to self "take first rank and are the most important duties of all" (*Collins* 27:341). But this statement only asserts a *philosophical* primacy of duties to self (Timmermann 2006, 509), not a blanket *normative* primacy of duties to self over duties to others. Kant's point, in a nutshell, is that we must comport ourselves in a manner appropriate to moral agents—to strive for moral goodness, remain good observers of duties, and acknowledge our moral equality with other rational beings (see Sect. 2.2). A person who does not do that at all would lack all moral worth and would also be unable to observe duties to others. By contrast, there is still hope for a person who observes duties to self but fails to observe duties to others (*Collins* 27:341). None of this implies that specific duties to self, such as cultivation duties, should take normative priority over other specific duties. We put the cart before the horse if we prioritise *cultivating* a capacity that can help us observe duties over the *actual observance* of our duties towards others. For instance, imagine that we can be crucially beneficent to a person by exploiting a piece of land, say by growing crops that help to save them from starvation. Clearly, we should not restrict our beneficence merely because the piece of land strikes us as sublime and presents a chance for us to cultivate our own capacity for aesthetic appreciation (see Chap. 10). The same is true, mutatis mutandis, for the exploitation of animals to the benefit of human beings. Whenever cultivating our capacity for sympathy would require that we do not make a certain contribution to another human being's happiness (perhaps by complicating their way of earning a living, by failing to cater to their gustatory preferences, by posing an obstacle to their customs, and so on), Kant cannot prioritise sympathy cultivation. So our duties regarding animals have little relative weight.

Once again, Kant's critics may be wrong about various details, but they are right about the general issue: Kant's account is too weak in its demands to match strong and common moral intuitions. The usual reaction to this insight is to reject Kant's account of animal ethics, or indeed all of Kantianism. Of course, the converse reaction is possible too: One can cling to Kant and deny or downplay the moral intuitions with which his view conflicts. This is a general weakness of arguments from intuition, and objections to the substantive upshots of Kant's view are no exception. Still, the discussion in this section has shown that Kant's account is severely restricted in what it can demand. This should show to traditional Kantians that they are not in the comfortable position suggested by much of the Kantian literature. To animal ethicists committed to the moral importance of animals, it shows that Kant's 'indirect duty' view is not a promising starting point for their philosophical case.

3.4   The Unhelpfulness of Kant's Account

To the structural and material objections discussed so far, let me add a more *practical* objection: Kant's account of animal ethics does not do what it is supposed to do. As I have explained in Sect. 2.6 above, Kant's moral philosophy is best understood as offering a certain type of *help* to ordinary moral agents. It helps us restore and refine our moral outlook in the face of our natural inclinations and their accompanying rationalisations. It shows that our ordinary feelings of moral obligation have a ground in reason and reminds us of the stringency of our duties (Sticker

2017). But when it comes to our treatment of animals, Kant's philosophy fails in exactly these regards.

The central move of Kant's account of animal ethics is to ascribe a confusion to ordinary moral agents, namely the 'amphiboly in moral concepts of reflection'. As mentioned before, Kant does not mean to say that ordinary agents are completely wrong about their duties in this area. They usually get the *content* of their duty right, he presumes: Do not be cruel or ungrateful to animals. Their only mistake is taking this to be a duty towards the animal rather than themselves. But then, what about agents who feel obligated to go above and beyond what Kant's duty of cultivation can demand? What, for instance, about people—vegans, vegetarians, and conflicted meat eaters—who cannot shake off the feeling that there is something wrong about killing and eating animals, a practice Kant himself explicitly condones (MM 6:443.16–17)? It appears that Kant must after all correct them. Such strong and far-reaching feelings of moral obligation towards animals, as widespread as they may be, have no ground in reason according to his view. But this clearly *undermines* trust in ordinary moral feelings instead of reinforcing it. Indeed, Kant fails to give reassurance to those who take their duties towards animals most seriously, to the vegans, vegetarians, and animal advocates who actually act on what they view as their duties to animals. This is disappointing, given that animal advocates' rationality is often questioned anyway (Wrenn et al. 2015). When it comes to animal ethics, Kant's moral philosophy fails exactly those real-world agents who could perhaps use its rational vindication most direly.

Kant's view is of just as little help when it comes to reminding us about the stringency of our duties, simply because cultivation duties do not demand very much and are unlikely to take precedent over other duties. As we have seen in Sect. 3.3, all that these duties straightforwardly demand of us is that we avoid adopting a practical-emotional stance that runs counter to capacities we should cultivate and that we adopt stances that cultivate these capacities. We should avoid cruelty for the sake of sympathy, ingratitude for the sake of gratitude, and lust for destruction for the sake of aesthetic appreciation. But this still allows most exploitation and mistreatment of animals, as long as it does not arise from a vicious stance. And where there is little to demand, Kant's moral philosophy cannot do much to remind us of the stringency of our duties more generally.

Finally, Kant's view fails to be helpful to contemporary ethicists interested in first-order normative questions. As we saw in Chap. 2, for the human domain Kant provides a whole taxonomy of duties. He distinguishes perfect from imperfect duties, direct from indirect ones, wide from narrow ones, and duties to self from duties to others. He provides an intricate account of the relation between happiness and morality, of inclination and duty, of free will and the moral law, and so on. And even if we zoom in on more specific moral questions, Kant has much to contribute, be it on lying, on beneficence, on friendship, on arrogance, envy, malicious glee, and so on. We find nothing even remotely comparable in Kant's account of the moral relations between human beings and animals. The rich taxonomy of our various duties towards human beings contrasts with a single type of cultivation duty regarding animals. Rather than a full-fledged system, here we find only one key claim and only one, barely fleshed-out argument. Kant's account of animal ethics fails to capture the complexity of our moral relations to animals as ordinary agents perceive them.

There are two important upshots here, one negative and one positive. The negative upshot is that Kant's account of animal ethics is not just structurally unsound, and not just too weak in its demands, but that it also fails to serve the main purpose of Kant's moral philosophy, viewed from a Kantian standpoint or the standpoint of a contemporary animal ethicist. On a sober look, this account is only a footnote to Kant's philosophical system, and not one particularly worth defending. Kantians and animal ethicists are much better advised to investigate ways in which animals can be properly included in Kantian moral concern.

The positive upshot, however, is that a tweaked Kantian system holds great promise for animal ethics. Kantian moral philosophy has a *point*. It clarifies, systematises, and vindicates an ordinary moral outlook, particularly for the strict moralists in the room. It enables us to understand more about ourselves and do some rich and challenging philosophy along the way. More than anything, it is this positive promise of a Kantian account of animal ethics that drives the present project. But clearly, if we are to reap these benefits, we must first find a way to include animals in Kant's ethical system.

To conclude, I have argued that critics of Kant's account of animal ethics are mostly right. The account is inconsistent, its demands are too weak, and it fails to be helpful in the ways Kant's moral philosophy is supposed to be. It just does not have a lot going for it. If we are more interested in animal ethics than defending a particular philosopher, we should abandon Kant's view once and for all. But at the same time, a Kantian system that incorporates animals more thoroughly avoids these pitfalls and holds great promise.

Acknowledging that Kant's 'indirect duty' account must go only reveals the bigger task ahead: We must develop some alternative. This will require that we get clearer on the reasons behind Kant's initial denial of duties towards animals. One idea will likely spring to mind for many Kant readers: It must all be about the Categorical Imperative. Human beings are ends in themselves for Kant, but animals are not. And it is only ends in themselves which merit moral concern for their own sake. Perhaps surprisingly, I do not think that this is where the issue lies. Moral concern, including duties towards individuals, is at stake in an entirely different part of Kant's ethical system. That is the topic of the next chapter.

REFERENCES

Aaltola, Elisa. 2012. *Animal suffering: Philosophy and culture*. London: Palgrave Macmillan.

Altman, Matthew C. 2011. *Kant and applied Ethics: The uses and limits of Kant's practical philosophy*. Malden, MA: Wiley-Blackwell.

Baranzke, Heike. 2005. Tierethik, Tiernatur und Moralanthropologie im Kontext von § 17, Tugendlehre. *Kant-Studien* 96: 336–363.

Broadie, Alexander, and Elizabeth M. Pybus. 1974. Kant's treatment of animals. *Philosophy* 49: 375–383.

Camenzind, Samuel. 2018. Der Paratext in Immanuel Kants Metaphysik der Sitten und seine (tier-)ethischen Implikationen. In *Tierethik transdisziplinär: Literatur—Kultur—Didaktik*, 43–59. Bielefeld: Transcript.

Carruthers, Peter. 2002. *The animals issue: Moral theory in practice*. Cambridge: Cambridge University Press.

Cavalieri, Paola. 2001. *The animal question: Why nonhuman animals deserve human rights*. Oxford: Oxford University Press.

Cooper, David E. 2018. *Animals and misanthropy*. New York: Routledge.

Denis, Lara. 2000. Kant's conception of duties regarding animals: Reconstruction and reconsideration. *History of Philosophy Quarterly* 17: 405–423.

Figley, Charles R. 1995. *Compassion fatigue: Coping with secondary traumatic stress disorder in those who treat the traumatized*. New York: Routledge.

Fischer, Bob. 2018. Arguments for consuming animal products. In *The Oxford handbook of food ethics*, ed. Anne Barnhill, Mark Budolfson, and Tyler Doggett, 241–263. Oxford: Oxford University Press.

Franklin, Julian H. 2005. *Animal rights and moral philosophy*. New York: Columbia University Press.

Frey, R. G. 1987. Autonomy and the value of animal life. *The Monist* 70: 50–63.

Gruen, Lori. 2015. *Entangled empathy: An alternative ethic for our relationships with animals*. New York: Lantern Books.

Hayward, Tim. 1994. Kant and the moral considerability of non-rational beings. *Royal Institute of Philosophy Supplement* 36: 129–142.

Herman, Barbara. 2018. We are not alone: A place for animals in Kant's ethics. In *Kant on persons and agency*, ed. Eric Watkins, 174–191. Cambridge: Cambridge University Press.

Hoff, Christina. 1983. Kant's invidious humanism. *Environmental Ethics* 5: 63–70.

Hsiao, Timothy. 2017. Industrial farming is not cruel to animals. *Journal of Agricultural and Environmental Ethics* 30: 37–54.

Kain, Patrick. 2018. Kant on animals. In *Oxford philosophical concepts: Animals*, ed. Peter Adamson and G. Fay Edwards. Oxford: Oxford University Press.

Kemmerer, Lisa. 2006. *In search of consistency: Ethics and animals*. Leiden: Brill.

Noske, Barbara. 1997. *Beyond boundaries: Humans and animals*. Montreal: Black Rose Books.

Nozick, Robert. 1974. *Anarchy, state, and utopia*. Oxford: Blackwell.

Otto. 1900. Ein fränkisches Dorf zu Anfang des 17. Jahrhunderts. *Zeitschrift für Social- und Wirthschaftsgeschichte* 7: 331–355.

Rachels, James. 1990. *Created from animals: The moral implications of Darwinism*. New York: Oxford University Press.

Regan, Tom. 1976. Broadie and Pybus on Kant. *Philosophy* 51: 471–472.

Regan, Tom. 2004. *The case for animal rights*. Berkeley/Los Angeles: University of California Press.

Ripstein, Arthur, and Sergio Tenenbaum. 2020. Directionality and virtuous ends. In *Kant and animals*, ed. John J. Callanan and Lucy Allais, 139–156. Oxford: Oxford University Press.

Rollin, Bernard E. 2011. *Putting the horse before Descartes: My life's work on behalf of animals*. Philadelphia: Temple University Press.

Schopenhauer, Arthur. 1915. *The basis of morality*. Translated by Arthur B. Bullock. London: George Allen & Unwin Ltd.

Sensen, Oliver. 2011. *Kant on human dignity*. Berlin: De Gruyter.

Singer, Peter. 2002. *Animal liberation*. New York: Ecco Press.

Sorabji, Richard. 1993. *Animal minds and human morals: The origins of the Western debate*. Ithaca, NY: Cornell University Press.

Steiner, Gary. 2011. Toward a non-anthropocentric cosmopolitanism. In *Anthropocentrism: Humans, animals, environments*, ed. Rob Boddice, 81–111. Leiden: Brill.

Sticker, Martin. 2017. Kant's criticism of common moral rational cognition. *European Journal of Philosophy* 25: 85–108.

Svoboda, Toby. 2012. Duties regarding nature: A Kantian approach to environmental ethics. *Kant Yearbook* 4: 143–163.

Svoboda, Toby. 2014. A reconsideration of indirect duties regarding non-human organisms. *Ethical Theory and Moral Practice* 17: 311–323.

Timmermann, Jens. 2005. When the tail wags the dog: Animal welfare and indirect duty in Kantian ethics. *Kantian Review* 10: 127–149.

Timmermann, Jens. 2006. Kantian duties to the self, explained and defended. *Philosophy* 81: 505–530.

Warren, Mary A. 1997. *Moral status: Obligations to persons and other living things.* Oxford: Clarendon Press.

Wolf, Ursula. 1990. *Das Tier in der Moral.* Frankfurt am Main: Vittorio Klostermann.

Wolf, Ursula. 2012. *Ethik der Mensch-Tier-Beziehung.* Frankfurt am Main: Vittorio Klostermann.

Wrenn, Corey L., Joanne Clark, Maddie Judge, Katharine A. Gilchrist, Delanie Woodlock, Katherina Dotson, Riva Spanos, and Jonothan Wrenn. 2015. The medicalization of nonhuman animal rights: frame contestation and the exploitation of disability. *Disability & Society* 30: 1307–1327.

Wuensch, Karl L., Kevin W. Jenkins, and G. Michael Poteat. 2002. Misanthropy, idealism and attitudes towards animals. *Anthrozoös* 15: 139–149.

Zamir, Tzachi. 2007. *Ethics and the beast: A speciesist argument for animal liberation.* Princeton, NJ: Princeton University Press.

PART II

Building Kantianism for Animals

CHAPTER 4

Is the Formula of Humanity the Problem?

4.1 Animals and the Formula of Humanity: Some Background

Despite their general unenthusiasm about Kant, many animal ethicists have adopted two pieces of Kantian terminology: 'being an end in itself' and its opposite, 'being a mere means'. Clark writes: "In my morality, all creatures with feelings and wishes should be thought of as ends-in-themselves, and not merely as means" (Clark 1997, 10). The "heart of human oppression of animals", according to Donaldson and Kymlicka, lies in "turning them into a means to human ends, rather than respecting them as ends in themselves" (Donaldson and Kymlicka 2011, 88). "Moral history will come to an end when all conscious creatures will enjoy the equal right to be treated as ends in themselves and not merely as means", says Kriegel (2013, 246). This vocabulary, adapted from Kant's Formula of Humanity (FH), seems particularly helpful to capture how animals are morally precious for their own sake, and how human beings often fail to respond to this preciousness.

However, it is exactly the FH which expels animals from Kant's moral universe in the eyes of most readers.[1] The formula asks us to "so act that

[1] Take, for instance: Wolf 1990, 34, 2012, 39, Warren 1997, 98; O'Neill 1998, 213; Regan 2004, 175; Korsgaard 2004, 2012, 2013, 2018; Franklin 2005, 39; Sensen 2011; Garthoff 2011; Cochrane 2012, 8; Kendrick 2012, 25; Cholbi 2014, 345; Kriegel 2013, 235; Grimm and Wild 2016, 37; Altman 2019. Overall, the view that Kant's exclusion of

© The Author(s) 2022
N. D. Müller, *Kantianism for Animals*, The Palgrave Macmillan
Animal Ethics Series,
https://Doi.org/10.1007/978-3-031-01930-2_4

you use humanity, whether in your own person or in the person of any other, always at the same time as an end, never merely as a means" (G 4:429.10–12). It is quite natural to assume that in the FH, Kant tells us *whom* we should treat *how*. Roughly: Persons, insofar as they share in a certain rational capacity or set of rational capacities ('humanity'), should be protected from harm and assisted in their endeavours for their own sake, not merely as a means to further, contingent ends. At any rate, on the popular reading of the FH, it is understood as a substantive moral principle which tells us how to treat individuals. To an advocate of the rights and liberation of human beings, the FH may appear like a very attractive principle because it seems so egalitarian. It appears to ground moral concern in capacities that, supposedly, all human beings share.[2] To advocates of non-human animals, however, the FH poses a straightforward problem: Whatever 'humanity' may be exactly, non-human animals most likely do not share in it.

If the popular reading of the FH is correct, Kantianism is inherently and inevitably inimical to the moral claims of animals. They are excluded from moral concern by the FH, which is a formulation of the Categorical Imperative, the supreme moral principle. So the popular reading that Kantian moral concern stems from the FH has important ramifications: It makes the exclusion of animals a core feature of Kantian ethics. Hence, Chignell calls the task of including animals in the FH "the holy grail among Kantian animal advocates" (Chignell 2021, 10).

But in this chapter, I will argue that there is an alternative to the popular reading on which the FH is a substantive moral principle that fixes the scope of moral concern. Indeed, it is hard to see how it *could* fix the scope of moral concern. On the reading I will suggest, this purpose is served by an entirely different part of Kant's ethical system, the doctrine of 'obligatory ends'. On this reading, Kantian moral philosophy is not as hostile to the claims of animals as many think. At least, any remaining hostility comes

---

animals from moral concern stems from the FH is often asserted or tacitly presupposed. To my knowledge, it has never been seriously challenged. Hence, it can be considered a standard view.

[2] Of course, *not* all members of the human species actually have the rational capacities Kant associates with humanity. Not all *homo sapiens* are moral agents, for instance. This makes Kant's ethical system vulnerable to the 'argument from species overlap' (see Sect. 2.1). For a detailed discussion on whether Kant can account for moral concern for literally *all* members of the human species, including small infants and certain people with disabilities, see Kain (2009).

from a different, more peripheral place in the system. Accordingly, including animals in the FH is not the 'holy grail' we ought to be chasing.

In my discussion, I focus on the FH, despite there being several other formulations of the Categorical Imperative.[3] I single out the FH for three reasons: First, in the literature it is standard to read the FH as expressing a requirement of moral concern (as Reath points out, Reath 2013, 210), more so than the other formulas. Secondly, the FH is often used to clarify the other formulas when their relation to moral concern is at issue (Wood 1999, 139; see also Franklin 2005, 39ff.). Third, the FH is the formula usually invoked to explain Kant's exclusion of animals (see footnote 1 above).

When we focus on the FH, the basic argument runs as follows: Kant's account of moral concern starts from the notion of humanity as an end in itself, and humanity—whatever it is—is an exclusive feature of finite rational beings. Therefore, there is no room for moral concern for animals, who are in the relevant sense 'non-rational'. To summarise, the argument at issue is this:

Exclusion of animals by the Formula of Humanity (FH)

(1) The FH and its supporting argument fix the scope of moral concern,
(2) and it draws the line precisely at finite rational beings,
(3) but animals are non-rational,
(4) therefore, animals must be excluded from moral concern.

Most readers take it that (1)–(3) adequately represent Kant's view and jointly explain Kant's exclusion of animals.[4] One response on the part of animal-friendly Kantians has been to argue *pace* Kant that (3) is false, usually by referring to empirical work on the cognitive capacities of animals (Rocha 2015; Balluch 2016; Thomas 2016; Judd and Rocha 2017). However, it is very hard indeed to argue that non-human animals are

---

[3] The standard reading counts four different formulas (Paton 1948). As Geismann (Geismann 2002) points out, however, Kant really offers twenty-seven slightly different formulations of the Categorical Imperative. Though they can reasonably be grouped together to yield Paton's four, it is generally worth remembering that Kant offers various formulas. Of course, this exacerbates the problem that Kant's formulas diverge in their moral guidance, if we understand them as substantive moral principles (a problem to which I return in Sect. 4.5 below).

[4] The philosophers listed in footnote 1 above all seem to endorse this view.

'rational' in the sense the argument requires. For 'rationality' in the sense
at issue requires transcendental freedom.[5] That is, animals would have to
be able to determine their actions independently of the laws of nature. But
first, this capacity is only possible through practical autonomy, through
acting on a self-imposed law. The empirical observations referenced in the
aforementioned contributions of course do not show that animals have
this capacity. In fact, no observation in the natural world, which is after all
structured by the laws of nature, *could* ever show that animals have the
capacity to determine themselves independently of these laws. And even if
we simply posited that animals are transcendentally free, this assumption
would counterintuitively imply that animals are Kantian moral *agents*.
After all, animals would then be capable of acting on an autonomously
self-imposed law, which in Kant's philosophy is the moral law. But if an
argument for Kantian moral concern for animals implies that animals are
Kantian moral *agents*, it proves too much. Therefore, rejecting premiss (3)
is not a promising strategy.

   A more popular response to the above argument is to dispute (2). This
is the strategy of two particularly influential voices in the debate: Wood
and Korsgaard. In Wood's view, the FH is fundamentally about expressing
reverence for the value of humanity. However, Wood argues, we can
express reverence for humanity even when dealing with beings who display only fragments or prerequisites of it, just as Christians can express
reverence for God in the way they treat his creation (Wood 1998, 197).
Therefore, Wood's view implies, the FH draws a fuzzy line which does not
strictly have to exclude animals.[6] Korsgaard argues that Kant's argument

---

[5] Consider, for instance, this remark in the second *Critique*: "For that [the human being]
has reason does not at all raise him in worth above mere animality if reason is to serve him
only for the sake of what instinct accomplishes for animals [...]" (CPrR 5:061.32–35).
Clearly, if we are going to equate "worth" (*Wert*) with the evaluative property that warrants
moral concern, then showing that animals possess reason in some sense is not enough. What
is necessary for an elevation in 'worth', in Kant's view, is that reason by itself can be practical,
that is, that the human being is free. My view, however, will be that this kind of 'worth' cannot, and is not meant to, account for moral concern for Kant.

[6] Admittedly, this is a somewhat simplified rendering of the position. Though Wood (Wood
1998) does argue that animals should be treated with respect in virtue of their possessing
prerequisites of reason, he also argues elsewhere (Wood 2007, 105) that no first-order normative injunctions follow directly from such basic principles without the addition of hefty
premises. The question whether humans may kill animals to eat them when other food is
available, say, is not a question that can be answered on the basis of fundamental Kantian
principles alone (ibid.).

for the value of humanity also implies the value of animality—of the capacity to pursue objects of choice. On her account, we must presuppose both these values in order to rationally follow our ordinary pursuits (Korsgaard 2004, 104, 2012, 14, 2018, 141–145). Therefore, the true line for moral concern is not to be drawn at rational beings, but at animals. Though Wood and Korsgaard certainly pursue a worthwhile goal in trying to include animals more thoroughly in Kantian ethics, there are reasons to be sceptical about the readings they presuppose in their rejection of premiss (2). I will explain these reasons in Sect. 4.3 below.

Yet another response is to agree with all of (1)–(3), but to conclude that the FH is therefore too narrow. Some argue that 'humanity' should be replaced by a more inclusive term such as 'sentience' (Franklin 2005, 35f.) or 'consciousness' (Garthoff 2011, 23f.). While this is a worthwhile and interesting strategy provided we believe all assumptions of the argument, it is not the strategy I intend to pursue in this chapter. For, in contrast to the previous literature, I am going to suggest that (1) is false. That is, I reject the tacit assumption that the FH fixes the scope of moral concern. The FH is, first and foremost, a principle describing the *form* of a good will (*how* a good will wills). It is not at the same time about the *material* of a good will (*what* it wills). But clearly, the question who matters morally—whom we ought to treat how—is a question about the *material* of a good will. For instance, whether a good will strives to make animals happy is a question about *what* a good will wills. This is just not the type of issue the FH, or any formulation of the Categorical Imperative, is meant to settle. My approach to the FH is not a completely new invention—it belongs in the already established camp of 'formal' approaches to the FH (Reath 2013). However, so far the literature has not realised the potential of such approaches for a Kantian animal ethic.

My argument rests on a distinction between *concern* (see Chap. 2) and what we may call *esteem*: a positive evaluative attitude towards beings which responds to their capacity to embody a good will. To use a metaphor, to have *concern* for someone is to reach out to them—to have *esteem* is to take one's hat off to them. These attitudes are distinct. The attitude of concern bears intimate connections to practical benevolence and more generally to our duties towards others. Esteem does not. This is an important distinction, since it is usually thought that Kant establishes the FH by way of an argument about the value that moral agents must necessarily ascribe to themselves. The trouble, in a nutshell, is that this self-ascribed value asks only for esteem, not for concern. And so the FH cannot provide a basis for moral concern. I follow up on this argument by showing how else Kant can account for moral concern, namely in his doctrine of obligatory ends. I then conclude with a brief statement of what the FH does, if it does not account for moral concern.

4.2   THE ESTEEM-CONCERN EQUIVOCATION

Recall the Kantian understanding of moral concern introduced in Chap. 2. On the conception I have proposed, moral concern is a matter of the duties we have towards individuals. Since Kant denies that we have duties towards animals, he excludes them from moral concern. Let us now turn to the central question: How does Kant establish that we should have moral concern for others? A standard idea among readers of the *Groundwork* is that Kant develops the requirement for moral concern for others out of an account of agency, or specifically of *moral* agency. "The rational nature exists as an end in itself",[7] Kant writes, and he adds: "The human being necessarily represents his own existence in this way" (G 4:429.02–04). The term 'end in itself' is standardly understood as a term related to moral concern—to be an end in itself is to be precious or to-be-protected in a special way (Reath 2013, 202). Hence, the idea seems natural that Kant bases moral concern on the following four-step argument:

The four-step argument for moral concern

(5) All and only rational beings necessarily represent themselves as ends in themselves.
(6) Therefore, all and only rational beings are ends in themselves.
(7) Moral concern is the appropriate attitude to ends in themselves.
(8) Therefore, all and only rational beings are due moral concern.

The key terms of this argument—'rational being', 'end in itself', 'moral concern'—have been interpreted in various ways in the literature. For instance, while some take Kant to be talking about 'rational beings' specifically in the sense of *beings who embody a good will* (Dean 1996) or who have at least "the spark of goodness" (Hill 1980, 87; see Hill 2009, 269),

---

[7] Here I diverge from Gregor's translation by adding the definite article. I do this because I believe that Kant intended the term "*vernünftige Natur*" to refer to the individual rational being, similar for instance to the German "*Frohnatur*" (as Timmermann 2007, 96, points out).

others take him to be talking more broadly about *beings capable of setting ends* (Korsgaard 1986; Wood 1999, 118). Due to such differences, the above argument captures not just one specific reconstruction of Kant's argument, but a whole family of reconstructions. What unites this family is that, in any case, the requirement of moral concern for rational beings is developed out of an account of agency viewed from the perspective of the agent.

What matters most for present purposes is what the term 'end in itself' means and how it relates to an account of moral concern in the substantive sense. In the following, I am going to argue that the four-step argument commits a fallacy of *equivocation*. Specifically, we mean one thing by the term 'end in itself' when we assert that rational beings necessarily view themselves as such, and we mean another thing by the same term when we claim that all such beings are due moral concern.

One reading which clearly drives a wedge between the premises of the argument rests on the claim that 'end in itself' is a *descriptive* term for Kant, as Sensen holds. On his view, Kant uses the term 'end in itself' to descriptively refer to transcendental freedom, so that 'rational beings are ends in themselves' is equivalent to 'rational beings are free' (Sensen 2011, 127–130). But if this term is purely descriptive, then there is no immediate reason why a being's falling under it would warrant moral concern for that being, as (3) claims. Indeed, Sensen notes: "Without freedom there would be no Categorical Imperative, but by itself this does not yet justify why one should respect others" (Sensen 2011, 107). So in order for (3) to be plausible, we would have to tacitly change the meaning of 'end in itself' halfway through the argument, committing an equivocation.

However, most readers take 'end in itself' to be an evaluative term, not a purely descriptive one (see Schönecker and Schmidt 2018). In other words, the term 'end in itself' denotes a kind of value. Because this is the standard reading, I will not pursue the argument based on Sensen's interpretation any further. However, even under an evaluative reading, the term 'end in itself' switches its meaning in the course of the four-step argument. In a nutshell, the problem is that the value we must plausibly presuppose ourselves as having *qua* (moral) agents is not a kind of value that plausibly demands moral concern for its bearer. To make this point in a more orderly fashion, let me expand the table of concern-related terms introduced earlier in Sect. 2.2 into Table 4.1.

There is now a new row of terms on the right-hand side, which lists counterparts to the terms previously introduced. While those towards

Table 4.1   Terms related to moral concern and esteem

	Concern-related terms	Esteem-related terms
Appropriate attitude	Moral concern	Moral esteem
Individual	Moral patient	Moral agent
Necessitation	Duty towards X	X's duty

whom there exist duties are called moral patients, those who *have* duties are called moral agents.[8] What I term 'moral esteem' is then defined as the appropriate attitude towards moral agents.[9]

Again, we can think of formal and substantive senses of each term, depending on whether we fill in specific duties or not. In either sense, however, esteem should not be confused with moral *praise*, which is after all only appropriate towards *good* moral agents. Moral esteem in the sense that matters here is appropriate even towards the scoundrel. In the formal sense, we can conceive of it as an acknowledgement and approval of the *potential* for moral goodness. This would presumably amount to an attitude of recognising that a moral agent is importantly distinct from all other things in the world with regard to her moral agency.[10] In a substantive sense, we can conceive of moral esteem as the approving recognition that an agent has the capacity and responsibility to fulfil a specific duty, say, to be beneficent.

[8] Let me add two asides about this terminology: (1) The dichotomy between moral agents and patients has been challenged in animal ethics (e.g. Rowlands 2012). This is not in tension to my point here, which is merely that there is a Kantian way to understand the received dichotomy. (2) Beings with a holy will—that is, a will which necessarily coincides with the moral law—do not count as moral agents according to the vocabulary I set up here. Angels and God may always do as the moral law demands, but in the absence of any inclinations that would lead them elsewhere, no *duties* arise. Duties are correctives for an imperfect will. Therefore, God and angels, although they can do good, do not count as moral agents in my vocabulary. Though surprising at first, this view should not be too awkward, given that we often take moral agency to be connected to the capacity to do *both* good *and* evil.

[9] A general difference between my vocabulary of 'esteem' and Kant's vocabulary of 'respect for persons' is that 'respect' refers to a *feeling* (see Sect. 2.1), while 'esteem' refers to an *attitude* (taking which may or may not be connected to a certain phenomenology). For this reason, I avoid equating 'esteem' with any of Kant's notions of 'respect'.

[10] This is what Sierra Vélez would call a recognition of human dignity (see Sierra Vélez 2020). To my mind, Sierra Vélez's distinction between 'human dignity' and 'animal dignity' maps well onto my own distinction between esteem and concern.

What is important to note now is that the terms in each column of Table 4.1 are *interdefinable* or *intensionally related*. The relations between the terms in each column can be stated correctly and straightforwardly in analytic claims. For instance, it is analytically true that moral patients are those towards whom there are duties. Likewise, to say that a person merits moral concern amounts to saying exactly that there exist duties towards this individual, or that she is a moral patient.

Having introduced this vocabulary, we can notice a gap which will have important implications for the four-step argument. There is a *semantic* gap between concern-related terms and their esteem-related counterparts: The contrasting terms in each *row* are not interdefinable. For instance, to say that someone merits *concern* is not merely a roundabout way of saying that they merit *esteem*. To say that someone is a moral *patient* is not merely a roundabout way of saying they are a moral *agent*. And to say that someone *has a duty* is not a roundabout way of saying *there is a duty towards* that person.

The semantic gap notwithstanding, a Kantian who endorses the four-step argument could say that the terms in each row stand in certain relations of *equivalence*, or even *identity*. For example, a Kantian can argue that moral concern is required towards exactly the same beings who also merit moral esteem, or perhaps even that the two terms refer to one and the same attitude at the end of the day. Similarly, the Kantian can say that all and only moral agents are patients, and that we have duties exactly towards those beings who themselves bear duties. At this point, we do not have to deny that any of this is possible. What matters, however, is that any such claims—be they about equivalence or identity, and be they true or false—are *not analytic*. They are *substantive* claims about moral matters. And because they are substantive claims, we can ask for substantive arguments in their favour, and these arguments can turn out to be fallacies.

Fallacies of *equivocation* are particularly easy to commit. What happens in such cases is that we use moral terms that can switch meanings between the left-hand and right-hand columns of the table. Take, for example, the term 'a person's moral value'. It is natural to take this as a term belonging in the left-hand column, as one semantically related to moral concern, patienthood, and our duties towards persons. To say that a person has moral value in this sense is to say that she is *precious*, to be treated with *concern*—think of Regan's term 'inherent value', for instance (Regan 2004, 241). Let us call this property 'moral value$_C$' to mark that it is intensionally linked to the notion of moral *concern*.

But of course, by the phrase "this person has moral value" we might also mean something else, namely that someone is 'a person of value'. This would most straightforwardly refer to the value of a good or decent person, and so it would be more closely related to moral praise than to what I have called esteem. However, it is also possible to understand 'a person's moral value' in the sense of 'the moral value of every person', as denoting an equal value possessed by all beings with the *potential* for moral goodness, even scoundrels. By stating that persons have value, we would then be saying that persons merit the recognition of their moral potential, simply due to their capacity to determine their will in a certain way (namely, independently of natural causes). Understood in this way, the term 'a person's moral value' is straightforwardly related to the notion of *moral agency*—let us call this 'moral value$_E$' to mark that this kind of value merits moral *esteem*.

Thus, the term 'a person's moral value' is ambiguous; it has several distinct meanings. This ambiguity alone does not need to trouble us. However, such ambiguous moral terms make it easy to commit what we can call the *Esteem-Concern Equivocation*. Consider an example:

The Esteem-Concern Equivocation

(9)   All and only moral agents have moral value$_E$.
(10)   All and only that which has moral value$_C$ deserves moral concern.
(11)   Therefore, all and only moral agents deserve moral concern.

This argument is fallacious. And it would not be any less fallacious if we put another ambiguous moral term in the place of 'moral value'—say, 'dignity'. Thus writes Herman: "If moral agency is a necessary condition of dignity, and dignity is what marks something out as a moral subject, then animals are not possible moral subjects" (Herman 2018, 178). It may be perfectly plausible to say that moral agents, and moral agents alone, have a 'dignity' and are 'beyond price', if by that we mean that moral agents have a potential for moral goodness that they should never decline to realise for the sake of non-moral goods like power, wealth, and health (see G 4:393.14). But if we claim in the next breath that this 'dignity' *obviously* demands that we protect others and promote their happiness, we have tacitly switched to a different meaning of the term, committing an equivocation. Nothing about the recognition of the potential for moral goodness *obviously* demands that we treat others with concern. What makes this equivocation particularly tempting is that its premises look very plausible, and in the case of (10) even analytic.[11] But equivocations do not generally make for good arguments.

Though they fail to be good arguments, equivocations are not beyond remedy either. The inference from (9) and (10) to (11) may be perfectly innocuous if we can supplement an additional premiss which links our crucial terms. There might be a convincing way to tie $value_E$ to $value_C$. We might claim, for instance, that the potential for moral goodness (associated with $value_E$) *makes* someone especially precious and to-be-treated-with-concern (in the sense of $value_C$). However, since 'esteem' and 'concern' are not intensionally related, this additional premiss is itself a substantive claim. Exactly this premiss would have been the crux of the matter in the first place!

Alternatively, a defender of the four-step argument could claim that the term 'a person's moral value' is not *ambiguous* but instead *multifaceted.* Whereas ambiguous terms have several distinct meanings (in the way the word 'triangle' denotes either a geometric shape or a musical instrument), 'moral $value_E$' and 'moral $value_C$' may refer to distinct *facets* of one and the same moral property, namely moral value. One could argue, for instance, that it is *exactly insofar as* an individual merits moral esteem that she merits moral concern—or even that moral esteem is *identical* to concern.

But mind the gap! The different facets of such a multifaceted term must themselves be joined together by a substantive background view. There must be some reason why the different facets can be meaningfully brought together under one label, why a blanket notion like 'moral value' is not a chimera. But then, a multifaceted term helps the argument no more than an ambiguous term. Both require a substantive background view to make the argument convincing. By way of example, consider again the term 'a person's moral value'. What is it about the potential for moral goodness—which has moral $value_E$—that demands that we treat a moral agent with concern? Why does this value give us a reason to be beneficent towards her, say?

The question might seem puzzling. It might seem obvious that no matter what kind of value we attach to whatever capacity, any valued capacity

---

[11] Premiss (1) is not analytic because it states that *only* moral agents have moral $value_E$. While it is analytically true that moral agents *do* have moral $value_E$, it is not analytic that *only* moral agents have it. Beings with a holy will, who do not qualify as moral agents (see footnote 8 above), might also have this kind of value.

and its bearer must be *protected* and the capacity's exercise must be *promoted*. That is enough to explain why moral value$_E$ leads to moral value$_C$. But it is not obvious by any means that all value demands this treatment. There are some evaluative attitudes and associated values which call for something else than protection and promotion. For instance, consider the value of what Kant calls the "terrifyingly sublime" (*Beobachtungen* 2:209.15). We may be in awe of a lion's capacity to overpower and maul a human being. This awe is an evaluative response, and it picks up on a special evaluative property of the lion's capacities. But of course, this should not move us to protect and promote the lion's exercise of this capacity. The terrifyingly sublime has a kind of value, but not a kind of value which demands protection or promotion.

Even in human interactions, there are cases in which we take a positive valuing attitude to some capacities of the other which does not make protection and promotion of those capacities appropriate. Take a game of chess: Here, valuing one's opponent calls for antagonism, not benevolence. I may approvingly acknowledge, even revere, my opponent's capacity to make her own moves in the present game, and I may value that she makes her moves rationally with the intention to win. We could even say that I value my opponent's instrumental-rational capacities in a categorically different, uniquely elevated way compared to, say, the way in which I value my knights or my bishops. After all, without a rational opponent, there would be no reason to value any of my chess pieces at all. But of course, valuing these chess-related rational capacities of my opponent does not make it appropriate for me to *let her win*. To the contrary, I display respect, reverence, esteem, and so on, by *restricting* her choices in the game as much as I can (literally bringing her into *Zugzwang*) and striving to end the game in my favour as quickly as possible. Hence, there can be valuings and values which call for actions diametrically opposed to the uninhibited exercise and the flourishing of her capacities. Of course, this is due to the inherently antagonistic nature of chess, and moral life is not like chess. But that is the point. There is some story to be told about why an individual's 'value' (or any evaluative property) demands what it demands. Values can demand various attitudes and actions, be it antagonism, noninterference, beneficence, or some other response.[12]

---

[12] To add yet another example, think of the antagonistic 'respect' some hunters profess for their prey. They recognise and approve of, say, a bear's intelligence and strength. They value these agency features on the part of the bear. But once again, the *way* in which the hunter

So we should not treat it as obvious that the distinctive value of moral agents demands that we treat them with concern in any particular substantive sense. Tying the unique value of moral agents to the value of what is precious and to-be-protected as part of a 'multifaceted' term—be it 'moral value', 'dignity', 'respect', or something else—merely shifts the question by one step, and this is just as uninformative as the equivocation we are trying to avoid.

Equipped with the idea of the Esteem-Concern Equivocation, let us return to the four-step argument:

The four-step argument for moral concern

(5) All and only rational beings necessarily represent themselves as ends in themselves.
(6) Therefore, all and only rational beings are ends in themselves.
(7) Moral concern is the appropriate attitude to ends in themselves.
(8) Therefore, all and only rational beings are due moral concern.

There are strong reasons to suspect that this is a token of the Esteem-Concern Equivocation, such that the type of value we ascribe to rational beings in (5) and (6) is one which demands moral esteem, but the type of value at issue in (7) demands concern. After all, (5) and (6) deal with a type of value which attaches to rational beings specifically in virtue of the way in which they necessarily represent themselves. It would be intuitive to interpret this as a value we ascribe to ourselves specifically as transcendentally free beings, a value that demands that we approvingly acknowledge the capacity of rational beings to act on a self-imposed law. But nothing in this notion of esteem for 'ends in themselves' suggests that we should have attitudes of practical benevolence towards others, or other attitudes characteristic of moral concern in a substantive sense.

There are two immediate objections to the hypothesis that the four-step argument commits an Esteem-Concern Equivocation. The first insists that (5) and (6) *already* ascribe to rational beings a type of value that

---

values the bear does not give the hunter any special reason to *assist* or *protect* the bear (which is why an animal advocate might object that this is not a morally valuable kind of 'respect' towards the animal). Doing so would in fact undermine the type of 'respect' at stake. This serves to show, once again, that certain types of valuing call for the inhibition and destruction, not the promotion or preservation, of the valued features and their bearers. Therefore, once again, the claim that valuing someone's agency features leads to a requirement of concern is substantive.

demands concern. This move would require us to read (5) as the claim that rational beings necessarily represent themselves as individuals who deserve moral concern. But at best, this is true for *human* rational beings as a matter of natural necessity, not of *all* rational beings as a matter of intelligibility. For instance, we can imagine rational beings who live in paradise, never requiring any beneficence from others. They would not have to think of themselves as beings who require or deserve moral concern, at least not in a substantive sense along Kant's lines. And even among actual human beings, there can very well be individuals who think of themselves as unworthy of moral concern—for instance, Kant's student and correspondent Maria von Herbert, who self-depreciatingly described herself as "superfluous, unnecessary" (Langton 2007, 160; see Wood 1999, 125). Hence, this objection fails, since it rests upon an implausibly strong assumption about what all rational beings necessarily take themselves to deserve.

One could also try to avoid the equivocation the other way around, by insisting that the moral concern in (7) and (8) is merely a function of the *esteem* we ought to have for rational beings. The most obvious way to make this argument is to say that, since we are talking about finite rational beings with needs and wishes, we must protect their life, needs, and wishes to the point that their distinctive rational capacities can come to fruition. One problem with this argument is that it has a hard time explaining why we should have concern for specific individuals, as opposed to a general attitude of maximising the exercise of valuable rational capacities, a sort of maximising utilitarianism of transcendentally free action.

Another, much more important problem is that concern (say, in the form of beneficence) does not generally make human beings more rational or free. Nor does it generally foster the moral exercise of their rational capacities. It may be the case that being too unhappy inhibits us from being good. This consideration leads Kant to accept that there is an indirect duty to secure a minimal level of happiness for ourselves (G 1.399.03 07, MM 6.388.17 30). But above a certain threshold of happiness, no strict correlation between happiness and esteem-related value exists. So why should we have benevolent or caring attitudes towards others if they are already above the threshold? Or why, to consider the opposite case, should we bother being practically benevolent towards those so far below the threshold that our beneficence cannot suffice to make them free? It would seem like we only have duties towards humans momentarily caught in a Goldilocks zone of debilitating, but not too debilitating unhappiness. This is absurd. Hence, we cannot plausibly insist that Kant's account of moral concern is merely a matter of protecting the conditions for the exercise of esteemed rational capacities.

The upshot of the foregoing considerations is that, even if we assume that 'end in itself' is an evaluative term and that the appropriate attitude towards rational beings is one of valuing their distinctive capacities, *we must not take it as obvious* that the distinctive value of rational beings is one which calls for moral concern. If we are not careful, we move illicitly from the assumption that rational beings merit moral esteem to the conclusion that they merit moral concern. To be sure, all is not lost. But if we are to move from the conditions of agency to a requirement of moral concern, we need a bridging story.

Two classic readings of the FH appear to provide such bridging stories, namely Wood's (Wood 2007) and Korsgaard's (Korsgaard 1986). What makes them particularly salient is that they offer detailed accounts of Kant's journey from the FH to moral concern. In a nutshell, Korsgaard develops an account of moral concern out of the view that we confer goodness upon our ends by choosing them, and Wood develops moral concern out of the notion of acting for the sake of humanity. I will explain why neither succeeds as a remedy for the Esteem-Concern Equivocation. In fact, they inadvertently repeat the same equivocation one step deeper into the argument. If we do not want to ascribe a fallacy to Kant, we should cease to understand end-in-itselfhood as the basis of moral concern, and we should instead pay attention to Kant's own way of accounting for moral concern elsewhere in his system.

4.3   Wood and Korsgaard Against the Esteem-Concern Equivocation

To repeat, to have moral concern 'Kantian-style' is to have an attitude relating to our duties towards individuals. Wood takes the FH to be central in the derivation of our duties, towards both self and others (Wood 1999, 135, 140f.). This derivation of specific duties works by means of a two-premiss argument (Wood 1999, 152f.). To use Wood's example of the duty not to give false promises (Wood 1999, 153):

Derivation of duties from the FH in Wood's view

(12) Always respect humanity, in one's own person as well as that of another, as an end in itself.

(13) A false promise, because its end cannot be shared by the person to whom the promise is made, frustrates or circumvents that person's rational agency, and thereby shows disrespect for it.

(14) Therefore, do not make false promises.

According to Wood, then, the FH accounts for moral concern. The FH provides all the normative force of the duty, while the "intermediate premiss" (ibid.) merely provides the subsumption of some specific action under the Categorical Imperative. Evidently, this gives the FH "radical import" (Wood 1999, 135).

Central to Wood's reading of the FH is the contention that it is a formula about *value*: "Though FH takes the form of a rule or commandment, what it basically asserts is the existence of a *substantive value* to be respected" (Wood 1999, 141). Wood's driving idea is that when Kant asserts that the human being "necessarily represents his own existence" as an end in itself (G 4:429.03–04), he means to say that in acting rationally, we already acknowledge the value of humanity (Wood 1999, 126). As he puts it elsewhere: "When it subjects my actions to rational guidance by an end, humanity [...] involves an active sense of my identity and an esteem for myself" (Wood 1999, 119). In setting an end for myself, the line of reasoning goes, I must presuppose that I am a being capable of picking out valuable ends. What we presuppose, as a referent of our valuing attitude of self-esteem, is the value of humanity as an end in itself.

It must be said that Wood's 'esteem' for humanity is not strictly the 'esteem' from our table in the previous section. According to Wood's conception, we have esteem for ourselves specifically *as agents*, not specifically as *moral* agents. Therefore, this notion of esteem is not so closely related to the notion of duty, but rather to the notion of end-directed action. What matters, however, is that there is still a semantic rift between *esteem* and *concern*, and this is all the more the case for Wood's notion of esteem.

Wood does not claim that esteem *equals* concern. However, he does believe that the esteem we have for ourselves *gives us reasons* to treat ourselves and others with concern. In Wood's terms, the value of humanity gives us "expressive reasons for action" (Wood 1999, 141). That is, the value of humanity demands that we act in a way that *expresses* the right evaluative attitude. As is well known, Kant emphasises the difference between an 'end to be produced' and a 'self-standing end', and he asserts that the end in itself is self-standing (G 4:437.27). Wood interprets this as the claim that the FH asks us to "*express* proper respect or reverence for the worth of humanity" (Wood 1999, 141). According to Wood's reading, then, rational beings are due moral concern because actions in line with moral concern express the right attitude towards the value of humanity.

Though Wood uses the term 'end in itself' uniformly, his reconstruction of Kant's account of moral concern still commits an Esteem-Concern Equivocation. The equivocation pertains to the notion of 'value' at issue. We may grant that acting on our ends already expresses a certain valuing attitude for our own humanity, since we presuppose that as rational beings, we are capable of identifying good ends. But it is unclear why the value we presuppose in ourselves should demand anything over and above *that we act on our ends*. Why do we not express reverence for others' capacity to choose good ends by leaving them to their own devices? After all, they will choose good ends even without our care or beneficence. So when we take it that reverence for humanity demands moral concern in a substantive sense, we have tacitly switched what we mean by 'value'. We started with a notion tethered to a kind of esteem, and we have finished with a notion tethered to concern. Thus Wood's Kant appears to commit an Esteem-Concern Equivocation, the ambiguous term being 'value'.

In Korsgaard's view, human beings *qua* rational beings are ends in themselves in the sense of being originators of valuable or 'good' ends:

> When Kant says: "rational nature exists as an end in itself. Man necessarily thinks of his own existence in this way; thus far it is a subjective principle of human actions" (429/47), I read him as claiming that in our private rational choices and in general in our actions we view ourselves as having a value-conferring status in virtue of our rational nature. (Korsgaard 1986, 196)

Korsgaard's central idea is that in setting an end, rational beings must suppose that it is good in the sense of being worth pursuing (Korsgaard 1986, 194). Indeed, our ends *are* good, but what makes them good is the very fact that they have been set by a "rational choice" (Korsgaard 1986, 196). Hence according to this view, rational beings are ends in themselves in the sense of being *originators* of the goodness of their own ends. This is why Korsgaard's reading is often considered to be 'constructivist'—goodness is here considered to be a feature brought into the world by the choices of rational beings. This contrasts with Wood's 'realist' reading, on which rational beings merely *presuppose* the existence of a substantive value, but do not themselves bring it into the world.

Now for the crucial step in Korsgaard's reconstruction: What is 'good' provides reasons for every rational being:

> the full realization and acknowledgement of the fact that another is an end in itself involves viewing the end upon which this person confers value as *good*—and when one acknowledges that something is good, one acknowledges it to be "in the judgment of every reasonable man, an object of the faculty of desire." To treat another as an end in itself is to treat his or her ends as objectively good, as you do your own. (Korsgaard 1986, 200)

Hence the fact that rational beings are ends in themselves has consequences for how we ought to treat them: We are to treat *their* ends as providing *us* with reasons for action. This seems like a mode of moral concern. Hence, Korsgaard's reading provides an explanation why 'being an end in itself' relates both to the distinctive capacities of rational beings and to moral concern.

However, now it appears that we have equivocated the notion of a 'good end'. In Korsgaard's view, the term 'goodness', as it is used here, refers to an end's feature of providing sufficient reasons for action (Korsgaard 1986, 194), but also of being "the object of every rational will" (ibid.). We can understand this as the claim that the ends set by rational beings provide 'public' or 'agent-neutral' reasons for action (see Korsgaard 2009, 191). That is, it is not merely the case that the end provides one particular rational being with reasons for action, but it is true in general that this end provides reasons for action to *any* rational being who has set it. An end's 'goodness', according to this notion, is its reasons-giving relation to any rational being who has set the end. But of course, no account of moral concern can get off the ground with this notion of goodness alone. As Godfrey-Smith points out: "You can have a respect for my good sense without being motivated to help me" (Godfrey-Smith 2021). What we need is not merely an end's feature of providing reasons to any rational being *who has set it*, but *to any rational being, period. Your* end should provide *me* with reasons, no matter whether I have adopted it. But then, the reasons provided by your ends must be 'public' in a much stronger sense.

One could defend Korsgaard by saying that she meant all along that the reasons generated by the ends of rational beings are 'public' in the stronger sense, namely in the sense that they exert normative force even over rational beings who have not adopted the end. After all, she puts great emphasis on the claim that good ends are "the object of every rational will" (Korsgaard 1986, 194). However, this turns Korsgaard's point into an argument we already dismissed earlier, namely that a rational being can only act under the presumption that she deserves moral concern in the substantive sense. This is patently not the case, as examples of self-depreciating people such as Maria von Herbert show (see Sect. 4.2 above).

Therefore, once again, we are left with two notions, one of which clusters with esteem and the other with concern. We may grant Korsgaard the claim that a rational being can only act on the presumption that her end provides reasons for any rational being who has set it, so that in a certain sense 'public' reasons must be in play. But when we go on to say that the goodness of our ends accounts for the requirement of substantive moral concern, we have taken a leap. We are now talking about ends that are 'good' in the sense of providing reasons even to beings who have not set them. Merely insisting that both are aspects of 'goodness' will not do— mind the gap. Otherwise we are merely reiterating the Esteem-Concern Equivocation.

To conclude, interesting and illuminating as they are, neither Wood's nor Korsgaard's reading of the FH gives a compelling account of Kant's journey from agency to moral concern. In the attempt to employ these readings of the FH to provide a bridging story, we have merely run into the Esteem-Concern Equivocation put in different terms. So the arguments which these readings ascribe to Kant end up being fallacious. Although one could always press philosophical arguments further, I take it that these difficulties are serious enough for us to consider an alternative reading of how Kant arrives at his conception of our duties to others.

4.4   OBLIGATORY ENDS: HOW KANT DERIVES DUTIES TO OTHERS

The way forward is to dispense with the popular idea that the FH encapsulates, or is very intimately related to, Kant's account of moral concern. One reason for this is that, as I have just argued, if we want to read an argument for moral concern into the passage leading up to the FH, that argument will not be very compelling. Another reason is that *treating individuals a certain way*, and so *treating individuals with moral concern,* inevitably has to do with effecting change in the world. To tell a moral agent how to treat individuals is to tell her what things to create, what processes to initiate, what states of affairs to bring about, in relation to those individuals. In Kant's terms, we are dealing with the prescription of *ends to be produced* (G 4:437.25). But as Kant makes abundantly clear, humanity as an end in itself is not an end to be produced, but a self-standing end (G 4:437.27). This should make us suspicious of any suggestions to the effect that Kant's account of moral concern derives from the notion of end-in-itselfhood.

However, there is yet another reason to disbelieve that Kant's account of moral concern is to be found in and around the FH: Kant provides a better account of moral concern elsewhere, in his doctrine of obligatory ends. The goal of the present section is to sketch Kant's argument for the requirement of moral concern. The last section will then be devoted to the question what the FH is there for, if not to provide a basis for moral concern.

When Kant introduces the notion of an obligatory end, he makes it clear that he is talking about *ends to be produced*: "An end is an object of free choice, the representation of which determines it to an action (*by which the object is brought about*)" (MM 6:384.33–34, emphasis removed and added). Kant then goes on to present arguments for two crucial claims: First, in general there must be an end that is also a duty. This is an end to be produced which we ought to adopt. Secondly, there are two obligatory ends in particular, namely one's own moral perfection and the happiness of others. These arguments jointly provide the basis for Kant's account of moral concern.

Kant's first argument is presented in a brief section of the introduction to the *Doctrine of Virtue*. Apart from the characterisation of ends as objects of choice whose representation determines action, Kant begins by explaining the notion of an obligatory end in more detail. He emphasises that "having any end of action whatsoever is an act of *freedom*" through which a rational being determines *herself* (MM 6:385.03–04). What is important here is that nature does not set *all* ends for rational beings (though it does set the end of our own happiness, see Sect. 2.3 above). Considered purely as rational beings, we are capable of setting ends for ourselves freely. The laws that govern the free setting of ends are a rational being's practical principles, not the laws of nature. Now the idea is that some principles command ends categorically, not merely as means to further ends. And an *obligatory* end, or "end that is also a duty" (MM 6:382.06–07), is an end that is commanded categorically in this way.

Having explained the notion of an obligatory end, Kant goes on to argue that there *is* indeed such an end: "Since there are free actions there must also be ends to which, as their objects, these actions are directed" (MM 6:385.11–12). Taken by itself, this only establishes that every free action has *some* end, not that there is one and the same particular end that is prescribed for every free action.[13] Kant however insists that "among these ends there must be some that are also (i.e., by their concept) duties" (MM 6:385.12–14). The reason for this is that autonomous action could not get off the ground without an obligatory end: "For were there no such ends, then all ends would hold for practical reason only as means to other ends; and since there can be no action without an end, a *categorical* imperative would be impossible" (MM 6:385.14–17).[14] The argument, as I see it, consists of two major parts: The first part is a view about free actions, namely that they exist, and that they are directed towards some end which is provided by practical reason, not by nature. The second part is a view about practical reason, namely that it determines action by means of principles which can either be hypothetical or categorical. Hypothetical imperatives have the form 'if X is your end, do Y' (see G 4:441.10–11), and hence practical reason can only use these principles to initiate action if some end (namely X) is already presupposed. Furthermore, since ends are often in turn means to further ends, hypothetical imperatives form chains or strings. These strings have to end somewhere if pure reason is to be practical; otherwise practical reason would merely be in the business of selecting means to presupposed ends. Now Kant's view, already established in the *Groundwork*, is that there is also a *Categorical* Imperative, which demands actions or maxims without reference to any presupposed

[13] If we were to take the premiss that all free actions have an end and conclude from it that there is *one* end of all free action, we would have committed an illicit quantifier shift. Of course, we should resist a reading that ascribes a blatant fallacy to Kant.

[14] Here I diverge from an influential reading in the literature, endorsed by Potter (Potter 1985) and Allison (Allison 1993). Potter and Allison both take Kant's argument to rest on the Categorical Imperative insofar as the Categorical Imperative expresses the moral law. They read Kant as arguing that the assumption that there are no obligatory ends leads us to the repugnant conclusion that there is no moral law, hence that there are no moral rules. By contrast, I read Kant as referring to the Categorical Imperative as the principle initiating transcendentally free action independently of nature. The Categorical Imperative is at the same time an expression of the moral law, but the emphasis here lies on freedom, not morality.

ends. Only thanks to this imperative is it possible for pure reason to initiate action at all. Hence, putting the two parts of the argument together, we get the conclusion that pure reason must supply at least one end of its own; otherwise it could not be practical. And if an end is provided by pure practical reason, that is an obligatory end. Therefore, there must be an obligatory end.

Kant concludes his section by emphasising again that the obligatory end is provided by reason alone, not nature. What matters for Kant's account of moral concern, however, is that he has set the stage for materially specific moral injunctions about what rational beings ought to do. That includes what they ought to do *to* themselves and others. Hence, the stage is set for moral concern.

The second argument Kant offers is that one's own moral perfection and the happiness of others are the obligatory ends. This argument is admittedly somewhat obscure, and the presentation is lamentably brief. On the face of it, Kant simply *posits* that one's own perfection and the happiness of others are obligatory ends without any preceding argument (MM 6:385.31–32). He does not seem to expect the reader to have any objections or questions regarding this point. However, his remarks in the following three paragraphs in the introduction to the *Doctrine of Virtue* do provide some basis for his claim.

Kant's strategy is not to argue positively for the claim that these two ends are obligatory, but instead to argue merely that the two converse ends—one's own happiness and the perfection of others—cannot possibly be obligatory ends. One's own happiness does not qualify as an obligatory end because it is "an end that all human beings have (by virtue of the impulse of their nature)" (MM 6:386.01–02; see Sect. 2.5), and "what everyone unavoidably already wants by himself, does not belong under the concept of *duty*" (MM 6:386.03–05). In other words, an obligatory end cannot perfectly map onto what we want as natural beings, or else it would lack its character of prescription. The problem with the perfection of others, by contrast, is that "it is self contradictory to require (make it my duty) that I ought to do something that no other than he himself can do" (MM 6:386.12–14). Kant's point is that perfection comes from setting moral ends and acting from duty, both of which we can only do for ourselves. It is therefore strictly impossible for us to promote the perfection of others. Though there are many small questions to ask about these arguments, we should focus on the big methodological issue: How is Kant's process of elimination supposed to work by which he determines the obligatory ends? How, in particular, did Kant arrive at the initial two candidates, perfection and happiness?

By and large, the consensus among Kant readers is that Kant derives the two candidates from his account of the highest good in the world (as Allison points out, Allison 1993, 18). The highest good in the world, Kant lays out in the second *Critique*, consists in complete virtue together with proportionate (complete) happiness (CPrR 5:110.31–111.05). Though it is not so clear in the *Doctrine of Virtue* that Kant is relying on this doctrine to derive the obligatory ends, he makes it quite explicit in the *Gemeinspruch*, published four years earlier:

> the need for a final end assigned by pure reason and comprehending the whole of all ends under one principle (a world as the highest good and possible through our cooperation) is a need of an unselfish will *extending* itself beyond observance of the moral law to production of an object (the highest good). (*Gemeinspruch* 8:279FN)

Kant's point here is directed against his fellow philosopher Garve, who had objected to the *Groundwork* that a will determined by a formal principle alone (in particular, a will that determines itself independently of all considerations of happiness) could never have an object, thus it would be indeterminate what a good will wills (Garve 1802; *Gemeinspruch* 8:278f.). In response, Kant explains that the good will 'extends' itself (*Gemeinspruch* 8:278FN) to include an intended product (though that product is not what gives the good will its moral worth). And Kant makes it clear that the way to find the intended product of a good will is to take the highest good in the world and leave out the bits that are unattainable through our actions (*Gemeinspruch* 8:279.19–22). This matches with Kant's process of elimination in the *Doctrine of Virtue*. Thus, it is reasonable to assume that Kant really does rely on his doctrine of the highest good in the world when arguing for the two initial candidates for obligatory ends.

At first sight, Kant's reliance on the doctrine of the highest good in the world poses a problem. On the one hand, the doctrine of the highest good is in itself a fairly controversial part of Kant's system. Allison remarks that it is "somewhat disappointing" to learn that Kant relies on the doctrine of the highest good to establish the obligatory ends (Allison 1993, 18). The greater difficulty for present purposes is however that Kant's conception of the highest good, both in the person and in the world, relies on the idea of "happiness distributed in exact proportion to morality" (CPrR

5:110.33). This would suggest that Kant must exclude animals, who after all never morally *deserve* their happiness in virtue of embodying a good will.

To my mind, there are two acceptable ways of resolving this difficulty. The first and stronger way has already been suggested in the literature: As Cholbi points out, Kant never claims that happiness is *not a good*, but rather that it is a good *conditioned* by morality (Cholbi 2014, 348). But happiness as a good is only so conditioned because it can corrupt the wills of human beings (ibid.). This is why Kant asserts that an impartial spectator could take no delight in seeing wicked people happy (G 4:393.19–22). But animals are crucially unlike wicked people. They cannot be morally corrupted by their happiness, since they are not moral agents in the first place. Though the happiness of animals is of course never *deserved* through virtue, it is also never *undeserved* through vice. In this way, their happiness is a more innocuous good than the happiness of human beings. If the highest good in the world is the greatest possible presence of goods (conditioned and unconditioned), then we should consider the happiness of animals to form an important part of it.

Note that this reliance on the doctrine of the highest good does not represent an endorsement of teleology (see Trampota 2013, 141). Good actions are still good in virtue of springing from a good will, not in virtue of contributing to the highest good in the world. Kant here uses the notion of the highest good as a heuristic or filter, as it were, to determine *what* a good will would want. It would want what any rational being could endorse as a good, which is the highest good in the world. But Cholbi's crucial point is that any rational being could very well endorse as a good the happiness of beings that are morally incorruptible.

The second way to resolve the difficulty is to circumvent the doctrine of the highest good in the derivation of the obligatory ends altogether. We can do this if we focus on the *practical* role of happiness and perfection as ends of human beings. In Kant's view, happiness and moral perfection are the *only* two ends human beings can pursue at the end of the day. In general, setting ends is a task of practical reason according to Kant (MM 6:385.01–04). It can accomplish this task in either of two ways: first, as pure practical reason, by supplying its own end; secondly, as instrumental practical reason, by choosing the means to the end nature has imposed on human beings, their own happiness. Practical reason implements these ends and means in action by means of practical principles, hypothetical or categorical. To repeat, practical principles interact in certain ways—hypothetical principles string together, so that each end is a means to a further end. Ultimately, human beings only ever act *either* for the sake of the end imposed upon them by nature, *or* for the sake of the end they set for themselves purely as rational beings. Insofar as human beings act from the ends imposed by nature, they aim for *happiness*. And insofar as they act from an end they set purely as rational beings, they aim for *moral perfection*. This argument then relies on Kant's background assumptions about human agency, but not about the highest good.

We can roughly summarise the proposed line of reasoning in the following argument:

Argument for the two obligatory ends

(1) There must be at least one obligatory end.

(2) Any end that a human being sets is in turn a means to either happiness or perfection.[15]

(3) Therefore, happiness and perfection are the two only ultimate ends (ends that are not means to any further ends).

(4) Obligatory ends are ultimate ends.

(5) Therefore, happiness and/or perfection are the only candidates for obligatory ends.

(6) *One's own* happiness and the perfection *of others* cannot be obligatory ends.

(7) Therefore, one's own perfection and the happiness of others are the only candidates for obligatory ends.

An obvious problem with this argument is that it cannot establish *that* our own perfection and the happiness of others are obligatory ends. It can only establish that they are the only remaining candidates. What is more, there is no guarantee that no further distinctions must be drawn, so that

---

[15] Note that the premiss here is not that human beings can act for the sake of happiness *tout court*, as opposed to *someone's* happiness in particular. We are inclined to promote *our own* happiness, and we can have a duty to promote *someone else's* happiness. The idea of acting for the sake of happiness *tout court* would be hard to accommodate in Kant's philosophy, and I thank Jens Timmermann for pointing this out. So the argument should be understood to begin from the premiss that human beings can only act for the sake of someone's happiness or someone's perfection, and to move towards the conclusion that only the happiness of others and our own moral perfection qualify as obligatory ends. As another side note, premiss (2) is a very strong claim. It implies, for instance, that human beings cannot intelligibly act for the ultimate sake of beauty, without that beauty being in turn a means to someone's happiness or perfection.

only *certain instances* of our own perfection are obligatory, and likewise only *certain instances* of the happiness of others. Indeed, Kant himself does introduce further specifications. He holds that it is only the happiness of others in the sense of their *permissible* ends that we ought to promote, not in the sense of their *impermissible* ends (MM 6:388.05–08).[16] Thus, the two obligatory ends do admit of further specification. What we can conclude from this reading is that the status of our own perfection and the happiness of others as obligatory ends has the character of a default status or a defeasible presumption.[17] The question we should ask now is not whether these ends *are* obligatory, but in which respects they *cannot be*. Hence what Kant achieves by the argument is not that he strictly *proves* these ends to be obligatory, but that he shifts the burden of argument.

How do we get from these two obligatory ends to moral concern? Moral concern 'Kantian-style', I have suggested, is an attitude of recognition of, and resolve to do, one's duties (or some specific duties) towards individuals (see Sect. 2.1). Kant's argument up to this point aimed to show that there are two obligatory ends, namely one's own perfection and the happiness of others. What still needs to be explained is how the obligatory ends lead to our *duties* towards self and others. To reiterate a point from Chap. 2, moral concern comes in formal and substantive variants. It can be recognition and resolve with regard to one's duties towards someone in general, or recognition and resolve with regard to some specific duties towards that individual. So the two questions we should ask at this point are thus: How do obligatory ends lead to duties 'towards' someone?

---

[16] Of course, this restriction is explained by the doctrine of the highest good. If what we ultimately aim for is complete virtue with proportionate happiness, we should not promote impermissible ends. Another way to account for Kant's view is to emphasise that happiness itself comes in a physical and moral variant (Kang 2015, 14). So to promote the happiness of others, we must take care not to make them objects of contempt in their own eyes, and so should not help along any of their morally impermissible endeavours.

[17] This conception of the two obligatory ends of course opens up the possibility that the happiness of animals is to be excluded from the obligatory end. I believe Kant implicitly advances just this claim on the grounds that animals cannot "constrain" us (MM 6:442.10–12). However, once we have arrived at a rough conception of the two obligatory ends, the burden of argument rests on the denier. This mirrors Kant's own method of providing arguments *against* one's own happiness and the perfection of others as obligatory ends. For this reason, I suggest that animal-friendly Kantians should disagree directly with Kant's argument that there can be no duties towards animals because they cannot 'constrain' us.

And how are we to derive the specific duties towards self and others which Kant thinks we have?

The first question—how we arrive at duties 'towards'—once again leads us into territory without consensus. But regarding this issue, there is also little debate. Here is my preferred reading. Kant does not explicitly offer a route that leads from obligatory ends to duties-towards. He appears to assume that we are already there. To repeat, obligatory ends *are* duties (MM 6:382.06–07). And Kant appears to conceive of them as duties *towards* self and others. That is, the promotion of one's own moral perfection *is* a duty to self, and the promotion of the happiness of others *is* a duty to others.

But assuming the obligatory ends are already duties 'towards' individuals, what makes them so? There are two basic explanations, both of which have a basis in Kant's writings. The first is that a duty 'towards others' is just a duty derived from the obligatory end of the happiness of others, and a duty 'towards self' is just a duty derived from the obligatory end of one's own self-perfection. Thus, the material of duty (the end we should adopt) determines whether it is a duty towards others or self. This fits well with the fact that according to Kant, our duties to self and our duties to others generally differ in what they demand of us. The second way of explaining the directionality of duties concerns the form or 'ground' of duty. Kant clearly adheres to the view that there can only be duties 'towards' those whose will, in a certain sense, "this constraint" us (MM 6:241.15–17; see MM 6:442.10). One aspect of this constraint is that the individual towards whom a duty is directed can always "release" the duty-bearer (MM 6:417.19). Therefore, if we ask whether the directionality of duties is a matter of the duties' material or form, Kant would answer yes to both. At any rate, the directionality of duties enters the stage together with obligatory ends, simply because these ends are already duties 'towards' someone. This gives us moral concern in the formal sense.[18]

As a preliminary upshot, Kant's account of moral concern for others (though not for ourselves) revolves around promoting happiness. To include animals in Kantian moral concern is to include them in this

---

[18] Of course, Kant's view that we have duties only towards those whose will 'necessitates' us presents a considerable problem to those of us who want to include animals in moral concern. I will deal with just this problem in the next chapter. To be upfront: I will argue that Kantians can simply reject the view that directionality is a matter of the form of duties, since it is already fixed by the material of duty.

happiness-promoting project in the right way. Although we have not yet considered in detail how the inclusion of animals might be achieved, we can already conclude that the line of moral concern can *at most* be drawn at the capacity for happiness. Animals who are incapable of experiencing hedonic states will inevitably remain excluded.

One can legitimately worry, however, if the obligatory ends comprise all we usually expect from Kant in terms of moral concern. What is often considered Kant's most important legacy in interpersonal ethics is the notion that others are not to be *treated as mere means*. How is this notion supposed to come out of the obligatory end of the happiness of others? Are we not rather left with a crude maxim of happiness maximisation? In the rest of this section, let me explore some things that follow from the doctrine of obligatory ends, and some that do not, regarding our treatment of others.

Among Kant's readers over the years, the notions of 'treatment as an end in itself' and 'treatment as a mere means' have taken on a life of their own, admitting of several popular interpretations. If we think of treatment as an end in itself as a treatment to which the recipient could rationally agree, given all information and sufficient time for reflection, then Kant's doctrine of obligatory ends gets us fairly close. It would certainly be in the patient's *best self-interest* to agree to the promotion of their own happiness—though perhaps it would still be *rational* for the patient to disagree with such treatment on moral grounds, since her duties are different from ours.

However, some interpretations of 'treatment as an end in itself' and 'treatment as a mere means' are more ambitious than what the doctrine of obligatory ends can give us. Take, for instance, the idea that the good of individual 'ends in themselves' must never be sacrificed for the aggregate good of many. In animal ethics, this absolute opposition to moral trade-offs is probably the idea most strongly associated with the labels 'Kantianism' and 'deontology'. Thus, Regan claims that "we fail to display proper respect for those who have inherent value whenever we harm them so that we may bring about the best aggregate consequences" (Regan 2004, 249). It is by no means obvious that so strong an idea follows from Kantian moral concern, understood along the lines I suggest. Moral concern as the recognition of our duties, and as the resolve to fulfil them, requires simply that we observe our duties. Certainly, our duties towards others rule out harming them *for the sake of our own happiness*, since our duty is to promote the happiness of others even at the expense of our own.

But to what extent it rules out sacrificing others for the happiness of *yet others* is a completely different question. In any case, we should not expect an answer to this question to follow from Kant's account of moral concern alone. If a prohibition of trade-offs is part of the Kantian picture at all, it must originate somewhere else in the system, particularly in his views on the resolution of (apparent) moral conflict.[19]

To summarise, Kant's account of moral concern rests on his doctrine of obligatory ends. The kind of substantive moral concern we get from Kant's account may be in the ballpark of some popular ideas about 'treatment as an end in itself'. Other ideas that are often associated with Kant do not follow, specifically a blanket prohibition of moral trade-offs. What is more, moral concern has only little to do with Kant's actual notion of 'ends in themselves'. Considered as objects of moral concern, we are *ends to be produced*. Things ought to be changed about us and our circumstances. In what sense we are 'ends in ourselves' is another matter, largely independent of our moral patienthood. At this point, one can legitimately wonder what the notion of an 'end in itself' is there for, if not to ground moral concern. Let me propose an answer in the following, final section.

4.5 What Is the Point of the Formula of Humanity, if Not Moral Concern?

So far in this chapter, I have rejected the popular idea that the FH is a solid basis for an account of moral concern. I have then addressed the worry that there is no other basis for moral concern in Kant by discussing the doctrine of obligatory ends. Another possible worry is now that my reading leaves the FH out of work. What, if not moral concern, could a principle be about, if it tells us to treat ourselves and others 'as ends in themselves', never as mere means? This is the topic of this section. My reading is only a variation over a theme already known from the literature. So my goal is simply to position my view in the debate and outline its main claims.

Reath (2013) has proposed a helpful ordering of different readings of the FH. On the one far end of the spectrum belong readings that see the

---

[19] Timmermann (2004) offers a less radical Kantian solution to conflict cases in which the concerns of the many are statistically more likely to decide what is to be done. For a general discussion of moral conflicts in Kantian moral philosophy, see Timmermann (2013).

FH purely as a substantive moral principle, usually a principle about moral concern. On the other far end stand those who read the FH purely as a 'formal principle', by which Reath means:

> the internal constitutive principle of a domain of cognition or rational activity. It is the principle that defines or describes and makes it possible to engage in that activity, thus the principle that any subject engaged in that activity must follow. (Reath 2013, 204)

When we read any formula of the Categorical Imperative as a formal principle, we view it as stating a constitutive rule of a rational capacity. As Kant points out in his overview of the different formulas (GMS 4:436.08–437.04), each formula emphasises a structural feature of the maxims of a good will: The Formula of Universal Law highlights that they have a certain form (that of a candidate for a universal law), the FH highlights that they have a certain matter (namely, humanity), and the Formula of Autonomy highlights that all these maxims stand in certain systematic relations to each other, forming a "realm" or "kingdom" akin to the realm or kingdom of nature structured by laws of nature. Thus, each formula points a spotlight at some feature of a good will, of practical autonomy. Kant himself claims that the Categorical Imperative "as such only asserts what obligation is" (MM 6:225.06–07).[20]

Now, Reath would strongly prefer a reading which brings together formal and substantive aspects of the FH (Reath 2013, 210). That is, he would rather interpret the formula as telling us *both* something about the nature of practical autonomy *and* how we ought to treat others. In his eyes, it is simply a desideratum for a plausible reading of the FH that it accommodates the "standard intuitive reading" of the FH as a substantive moral principle about concern (Reath 2013, 208). However, if we appreciate what the doctrine of obligatory ends does for Kant's account of moral concern, we simply do not *need* the FH to be a substantive moral principle. If we want, we are free to understand the FH and the other formulas as purely formal principles of practical autonomy, with all the substantive action-guidance being provided by the doctrine of obligatory ends later on.

---

[20] Here I have replaced Gregor's "affirms" with "asserts". It appears more straightforward as a translation for Kant's "*aussagt*" (MM 6:225.06). I take Kant to say that the Categorical Imperative tells us (asserts) what moral obligation or necessitation ('*Verbindlichkeit*') consists in.

So what does the FH tell us about practical autonomy? Recall the main formulation of the FH: "So act that you use humanity, whether in your own person or in the person of any other, always at the same time as an end, never merely as a means" (G 4:429.10–12). The term 'humanity', I take it, refers to a rational being's capacity to act on a self-imposed law, rather than merely according to natural laws. This is practical autonomy, and the self-imposed law is the moral law. What the FH tells us, in a nutshell, is that we must take this capacity itself into view if we are to exercise it.

This is not to say that we must simply *contemplate* autonomy or the moral law in order to act autonomously. Rather, we must have autonomy in view *as an end*—an object with regard to which we determine our action (see MM 6:381.04–06). To be sure, it is not an end like any other. Many of our ordinary ends are external things we aim to produce through our actions. For instance, I might use the coffee maker as a means, a cup of coffee being my end. Unlike the future cup of coffee, autonomy is neither external to the agent nor is it a yet non-existent thing. It is already there and inherent in the very type of end-setting at issue. It is not an 'end to be produced' (G 4:437.26–27). Still, autonomy is an 'end' in the more general sense of an object with regard to which our action is determined. Of course, any particular maxim of a good will also has an end to be produced—for example, the happiness of some particular person, or the cultivation of some of the agent's own capacities that are serviceable to morality. But if we want to know more about these kinds of ends of a good will, we should not consult the FH, but the doctrine of obligatory ends. On the purely formal reading, the FH tells us *something* about one kind of end of a good will, but not *everything* about *all* kinds of ends it adopts.

Kant's point, as I read it, is that we can only act autonomously if we take autonomy into view as an end, namely by setting out to *exercise autonomy well*. Autonomy is the capacity to act on a self-imposed moral law. This capacity comes with its own standard, namely the moral law itself. And so we exercise autonomy *well* only if we set out to *follow* the moral law. So to treat humanity as an end, in effect, is to strive to follow the moral law. By contrast, to use humanity as a mere means is to use the capacity to act on a self-imposed law for any other purpose than to actually *follow* that law.

Here is a good place to provide an example, and the obvious choice is Kant's case from the *Groundwork*, the prohibition of prudential suicide. Kant imagines a man who is "someone who has suicide in mind" (G 4:429.16). In other words, this person is *considering* suicide. He is not acting on blind impulse but contemplating different ends which he could adopt. Some of these ends stem from nature, and others from reason. The opposition, it is quite clear for Kant, is one between inclination-based ends which demand suicide (to avoid greater future suffering) and ends autonomously set by pure reason which demand continuing an unpleasant life (in order to remain capable of fulfilling one's duties). The man who contemplates suicide is aware of this opposition. But in order merely to *contemplate* the ends he could adopt from pure reason, the man has already had to impose the moral law on himself. He can *cognise* the moral law only by *self-imposing* it. And so he must *do* what the moral law demands, which is to refrain from suicide. Beings with the capacity to act on a self-imposed moral law must strive to exercise this capacity well, to actually follow the moral law. To contemplate the options and then do what inclinations demand is to use the capacity merely as a means for our own happiness. This is what the example illuminates.

To be sure, Kant's discussion of the four *Groundwork* examples also presents some difficulties for a purely formal reading. First, Kant also speaks of *human beings* as ends in themselves, not just humanity (e.g. MM 6:429.03–04; MM 6:429.20–23). This is somewhat misleading. Evidently, what Kant here means by 'human beings' are individuals *insofar as they are capable of acting on a self-imposed law*. At the end of the day, it is more straightforward to say *of the capacity* that it is an end in itself (that we must strive to exercise it well). To say the same of the *bearer* of the capacity is merely derivative.

A second problem is more serious: Kant also talks about humanity in the person of *others*. It too should be treated as an end in itself, never as a mere means. In general, I understand this as an emphasis on the fact that humanity as a capacity is not tied to particular individuals but is the same capacity in all autonomous beings. However, it cannot be denied that Kant himself appears to read an awful lot into the notion of treating others' humanity as an end in itself, especially in his discussion of false promises. He seamlessly begins to comment on whether others "can contain" the same end and takes this as a marker of whether humanity is being treated as an end (G 4:429f.). What is going on?

On my preferred reading, Kant is taking a detour here for the sake of adding some variety to the discussion. His overall goal in the examples is, still, to illustrate an aspect of morality using examples of obvious immorality. The situation in the false promise example is, once again, someone who *contemplates* different actions, one of which is giving a false promise in order to obtain some money. As in the case of prudential suicide, what should be shown is that in using autonomy to contemplate options, Kant's agent already subjects himself to the moral law. Humanity is inherently a capacity to be exercised *well*. So Kant could simply repeat his point from the suicide example: Autonomy inherently demands that we follow the moral law. And the agent in the example already knows what the moral law demands, namely not to make a false promise. In other words, Kant could also have emphasised that the lying promiser is using humanity *in his own person* as a mere means.

Instead, however, Kant chooses to emphasise humanity in the person on the receiving end of the action. I suggest his move is the following: A will who exercises autonomy *well* sets an end from pure reason, in accordance with the moral law. And if an end is set from pure reason, any rational being in any natural circumstances could have set it. This even includes those who stand to be harmed by the proposed action, such as the recipient of the false promise. That this person could not have set the same end shows that the false promiser's end cannot be set from pure reason. It must be set from inclination. And so by contemplating his options and opting for an inclination-based end, he has failed to treat humanity as an end in itself.

Although Kant's discussion of the four examples puts a purely formal reading of the FH to the test, formal readings also come with a general advantage: As Reath points out (Reath 2013, 224), formal readings make it much easier to account for the equivalence of the different formulations of the Categorical Imperative. The problem is familiar in the Kantian literature that the various formulas appear to give divergent moral guidance if we interpret them as substantive principles (Geiger 2015). It would appear as if the Formula of Universal Law, the Formula of the Law of Nature, the FH, and the Formula of Autonomy all make divergent substantive prescriptions, so that cases abound in which some formulas are observed, but not others. Formal readings avoid this difficulty altogether, since each of the formulas contains no substantive moral guidance from which the others could diverge.

What about Kant's argument that every rational being inevitably views her own existence as an end in itself? To cut a long story short, I want to suggest we are not truly dealing with an argument here. Kant is making a comment about the reflexivity of pure practical reason. In the passage leading up to the FH, Kant asserts about the Categorical Imperative: "The ground of this principle is: *the rational nature exists as an end in itself.* The human being necessarily represents his own existence in this way" (G 4:429.02–04). Now if we interpret the term 'end in itself' along the lines I suggest, Kant is saying that any rational being views her own autonomy as a self-standing end—something to be used *well*, by its own inherent standard, which is the moral law. Therefore, Kant's comment simply states that we already regard our own autonomy as tied to the moral law.

Kant then adds that "every other rational being also represents his existence in this way consequent on just the same rational ground that also holds for me" (G 4:429.05–07). To this he attaches a footnote that has puzzled many readers: "Here I put forward this proposition as a postulate. The grounds for it will be found in the last Section" (G 4:429FN). Why does Kant think he has not supported his assertion enough? The answer is that up to this point, Kant has only asserted that the rational being, from a first-person standpoint, takes her autonomy to be tied to the moral law. The capacity to act on a self-imposed law rather than merely natural laws always *presents itself to us* as something to be used *well*. But it could *present* itself thus even if morality were a mere phantom or chimera (G 4:445.08). The assertion Kant then makes, namely that myself and other rational beings *have a rational ground* for viewing our own autonomy in this way, is stronger. This stronger assertion requires that we show that morality is not a chimera, that we can indeed act on a moral law as opposed to natural laws. We must show, in other words, that the will really is free. And that is what Kant sets out to show later, as promised, in *Groundwork III*.

To summarise, on my preferred reading, the FH is a purely formal principle of autonomous willing. It tells us that as soon as we exercise our capacity to act on a self-imposed law in any way, we are bound to exercise it well, thus to actually follow the moral law. As soon as we use this capacity to another end than to follow the moral law, we use it as a mere means. Thus we fail by a standard already internal to autonomous willing itself. To be sure, this section has not shown that *only* a purely formal reading of the FH can be coherent and fruitful—just that it too can be. Adopting a purely formal reading of the FH shifts our perspective away from the question whether animals are 'ends in themselves' and towards the question whether their happiness should be considered a part of the obligatory end of the happiness of others. This is the kind of reading we need in order to include animals in Kantian moral concern.

Between Kant and today's animal advocates, there are some disagreements. What they need *not* quarrel about, however, is the FH. Contrary to popular opinion, I have argued that the FH cannot be the basis for moral concern that many take it to be. The problem is that the substantive value the FH would establish (if it were to establish any) would have to emerge out of the conditions of agency—out of how "[the] human being necessarily represents his own existence" (G 4:429.02–04). But even if we grant that human beings ascribe to themselves some substantive value, it cannot be a value that accounts for moral concern. The value will demand that we have *esteem* for the agent. But this is not the same as demanding *concern*. We can take our hat off to someone, and even be in awe of their capacity to act from the moral law, but still see no reason whatsoever to reach out to them with moral concern. The influential readings by Wood and Korsgaard cannot bridge this gap without equivocating esteem- and concern-related terms further down the line.

I have offered an alternative account both of how Kant arrives at moral concern and of what the FH is there for. Kant establishes moral concern with his doctrine of obligatory ends. The two obligatory ends are one's own moral perfection and the happiness of others. All of our materially specific duties are derived from these ends. The philosophically crucial moves lie in establishing that there must be obligatory ends at all and that they are specifically the two ends Kant mentions. If we grant Kant these moves, however, moral concern is established. The FH ends up playing no special role for moral concern. Its purpose is entirely different and lies in illuminating the good will. In a nutshell, the FH tells us that autonomous willing inherently calls for the observance of the moral law. Humanity is the capacity to act on a self-imposed law, and we can only exercise this capacity if we reflectively take it into view (treat it as an end of our action) by striving to exercise it *well*. This requires that we set out to actually follow the moral law. We must not use our humanity merely to contemplate possible options and then go with what our inclinations favour. On this reading, the FH is a formal principle of an autonomous will, not a substantive principle about moral concern.

The main move of this chapter has been to set an issue aside. It may seem as though this is a mere preliminary to the real discussion, and in a way it is. But this preliminary is important. At the end of the day, the question at stake here is whether the exclusion of animals from moral concern follows from the very core of Kant's ethical system. The FH is, after all, a formula of the Categorical Imperative, the supreme moral principle. The most important message of this chapter is thus: No, the exclusion of animals is *not* a necessary feature of the supreme Kantian moral principle. The issue lies elsewhere.

REFERENCES

Allison, Henry E. 1993. Kant's doctrine of obligatory ends. *Jahrbuch für Recht und Ethik* 1: 7–24.

Altman, Matthew C. 2019. Animal suffering and moral salience: A defense of Kant's indirect view. *The Journal of Value Inquiry* 53: 275–288.

Balluch, Martin. 2016. Autonomie bei Hunden: Die Fähigkeit, das eigene Handeln durch selbst gesetzte Zwecke Regeln zu unterwerfen, macht nichtmenschliche Tiere im Kant'schen Sinne zu Zwecken an sich. In *Das Handeln der Tiere: Tierliche Agency im Fokus der Human-Animal Studies*, ed. Sven Wirth, Anett Laue, Markus Kurth, Katharina Dornenzweig, Leonie Bossert, and Karsten Balgar, 203–225. Bielefeld: Transcript.

Chignell, Andrew. 2021. Fellow creatures: Our obligations to the other animals, by Christine M. Korsgaard. *Mind* 130: 363–373.

Cholbi, Michael. 2014. A direct Kantian duty to animals. *The Southern Journal of Philosophy* 52: 338–358.

Clark, Stephen R. L. 1997. *Animals and their moral standing*. London: Routledge.

Cochrane, Alasdair. 2012. Animal rights without liberation: Applied ethics and human obligations. New York: Columbia University Press.

Dean, Richard. 1996. What should we treat as an end in itself? *Pacific Philosophical Quarterly* 77: 268–288.

Donaldson, Sue, and Will Kymlicka. 2011. *Zoopolis: A political theory of animal rights*. New York: Oxford University Press.

Franklin, Julian H. 2005. *Animal rights and moral philosophy*. New York: Columbia University Press.

Garthoff, Jon. 2011. Meriting concern and meriting respect. *Journal of Ethics & Social Philosophy* 5: 1–28.

Garve, Christian. 1802. *Versuche über verschiedene Gegenstände aus der Moral, der Litteratur und dem gesellschaftlichen Leben*. Breslau: Korn.

Geiger, Ido. 2015. How are the different formulas of the Categorical Imperative related? *Kantian Review* 20: 395–419.

Geismann, Georg. 2002. Die verschiedenen Formeln des kategorischen Imperativs. *Kant-Studien* 93: 374–384.

Godfrey-Smith, Peter. 2021. Philosophers and other animals. *Aeon*.

Grimm, Herwig, and Markus Wild. 2016. *Tierethik zur Einführung*. Hamburg: Junius.

Herman, Barbara. 2018. We are not alone: A place for animals in Kant's ethics. In *Kant on persons and agency*, ed. Eric Watkins, 174–191. Cambridge: Cambridge University Press.

Hill, Thomas E. 1980. Humanity as an end in itself. *Ethics* 91: 84–99.

Hill, Thomas E., ed. 2009. *The Blackwell guide to Kant's ethics*. Malden, MA: Wiley-Blackwell.

Judd, David, and James Rocha. 2017. Autonomous pigs. *Ethics and the Environment* 22: 1–18.

Kain, Patrick. 2009. Kant's defense of human moral status. *Journal of the History of Philosophy* 47: 59–101.
Kang, Ji-Young. 2015. Die allgemeine Glückseligkeit: Zur systematischen Stellung und Funktionen der Glückseligkeit bei Kant. Berlin: De Gruyter.
Kendrick, Heather M. 2012. A place for animals in the Kingdom of Ends. In *Strangers to nature: Animal lives and human ethics*, ed. Gregory R. Smulewicz-Zucker, 35–65. Lanham, MD: Lexington Books.
Korsgaard, Christine M. 1986. Kant's Formula of Humanity. *Kant-Studien* 77: 183–202.
Korsgaard, Christine M. 2004. Fellow creatures. The Tanner Lectures on Human Values.
Korsgaard, Christine M. 2009. *Self-constitution: Agency, identity, and integrity.* Oxford: Oxford University Press.
Korsgaard, Christine M. 2012. A Kantian case for animal rights. In *Animal law – Tier und Recht: Developments and perspectives in the 21st century*, ed. Margot Michel, Daniela Kühne, and Julia Hänni, 3–25. Zürich/St. Gallen: DIKE.
Korsgaard, Christine M. 2013. Kantian ethics, animals, and the law. *Oxford Journal of Legal Studies* 33: 629–648.
Korsgaard, Christine M. 2018. *Fellow creatures: Our obligations to the other animals.* Oxford: Oxford University Press.
Kriegel, Uriah. 2013. Animal rights: A non-consequentialist approach. In *Animal minds and animal ethics: Connecting two separate fields*, ed. Klaus Petrus and Markus Wild, 231–247. Bielefeld: Transcript.
Langton, Rae. 2007. Objective and unconditioned value. *Philosophical Review* 116: 157–185.
O'Neill, Onora. 1998. Kant on duties regarding nonrational nature – necessary anthropocentrism and contingent speciesism. *Aristotelian Society Supplementary Volume* 72: 211–228.
Paton, Herbert J. 1948. The Categorical Imperative: A study in Kant's moral philosophy. London: Hutchinson.
Potter, Nelson. 1985. Kant on ends that are at the same time duties. *Pacific Philosophical Quarterly* 66: 78–92.
Reath, Andrews. 2013. Formal approaches to Kant's Formula of Humanity. In *Kant on practical justification*, ed. Mark Timmons and Sorin Baiasu, 201–228. Oxford: Oxford University Press.
Regan, Tom. 2004. *The case for animal rights.* Berkeley/Los Angeles: University of California Press.
Rocha, James. 2015. Kantian respect for minimally rational animals. *Social Theory and Practice* 41: 309–327.
Rowlands, Mark. 2012. *Can animals be moral?* Oxford: Oxford University Press.
Schönecker, Dieter, and Elke Schmidt. 2018. Kant's ground-thesis. On dignity and value in the groundwork. *The Journal of Value Inquiry* 52: 81–95.
Sensen, Oliver. 2011. *Kant on human dignity.* Berlin: De Gruyter.

Sierra Vélez, Lucas. 2020. The dignity of person: Kantian ethics and utilitarianism. Doctoral dissertation, University of St Andrews.

Thomas, Natalie. 2016. *Animal ethics and the autonomous animal self.* New York: Palgrave Macmillan.

Timmermann, Jens. 2004. The individualist lottery: How people count, but not their numbers. *Analysis* 64: 106–112.

Timmermann, Jens. 2007. *Kant's Groundwork of the Metaphysics of Morals: A commentary.* Cambridge: Cambridge University Press.

Timmermann, Jens. 2013. Kantian dilemmas? Moral conflict in Kant's ethical theory. *Archiv für Geschichte der Philosophie* 95: 2013.

Trampota, Andreas. 2013. The concept and necessity of an end in ethics (TL 6:379–389). In *Kant's "Tugendlehre": A comprehensive commentary*, ed. Andreas Trampota, Oliver Sensen, and Jens Timmermann, 139–157. Berlin: De Gruyter.

Warren, Mary A. 1997. Moral status: Obligations to persons and other living things. Oxford: Clarendon Press.

Wolf, Ursula. 1990. *Das Tier in der Moral.* Frankfurt am Main: Vittorio Klostermann.

Wolf, Ursula. 2012. *Ethik der Mensch-Tier-Beziehung.* Frankfurt am Main: Vittorio Klostermann.

Wood, Allen W. 1998. Kant on duties regarding non-rational nature. *Aristotelian Society Supplementary Volume* 72: 189–210.

Wood, Allen W. 1999. *Kant's ethical thought.* Cambridge: Cambridge University Press.

Wood, Allen W. 2007. *Kantian ethics.* Cambridge: Cambridge University Press.

CHAPTER 5

Animals and the 'Directionality' of Duties

5.1   Do We Truly 'Share' the Moral Law? Thompson's Challenge to Kant

Kant ties the notion of a 'duty towards someone' to the idea of 'necessitat-ing' or 'constraining' one another under the moral law (MM 6:442.10; see also MM 6:241.15–17). This is his stated reason for restricting moral status to persons, excluding animals (MM 6:442.11–12). Although Kant never makes explicit what this 'constraining' activity consists in, it is clear from the context that only individuals who *mutually share the moral law* can constrain each other in this way (MM 6:442.11–12; Wood 1998, 189; Korsgaard 2018, 123ff.; Ripstein and Tenenbaum 2020, 147). So when it comes to the conditions of the possibility of duties towards others, the animal advocate has a bone to pick with Kant.

In this chapter I propose a way to amend Kant's conception of moral duties so that moral duties can be directed towards animals. For my argu-ment, I enlist some outside help from critics who object that moral agents, as Kant conceives of them, cannot genuinely *share* the moral law in the first place. Thompson (2004) has argued that since the moral law is auton-omous, individual Kantian agents stand under *separate moral laws with the same content each*, but not under *one and the same, shared moral law*. The upshot for Thompson is that Kant quite simply fails to account for the directionality of duties. The usual Kantian reaction has been to come up with an account of how the moral law is shared between Kantian persons

© The Author(s) 2022
N. D. Müller, *Kantianism for Animals*, The Palgrave Macmillan
Animal Ethics Series,
https://doi.org/10.1007/978-3-031-01930-2_5

after all (Fanselow 2008; Darwall 2009; Palatnik 2018). For reasons I will explain in this chapter, this is not my preferred response. I argue that we can, and should, account for directionality in an entirely different way and that Kant provides all the resources we need.

In a nutshell, I suggest we should account for directionality in terms of the *content* of our duties. Duties towards others are just duties that are *about others* in a certain special way. Likewise, duties towards self are just duties that are *about ourselves* in a certain special way. But of course, duties can be *about* others even if those others do not share the moral law. So with my conception of directionality, I remove any elements of what today's ethicists sometimes call 'second-personal ethics' from Kant's system. What remains is a version of Kant's ethics that doubles down on the "fundamentally and radically first-personal" features it already has (Timmermann 2014, 131; see also Sensen 2011, 120f.). I suggest it is all the better for it, certainly from the perspective of an animal ethicist. On the 'first-personal' conception of directionality, there can very well be duties towards animals, and they do not categorically differ in form or ground from our duties towards other human beings.

To approach the notion of directionality, consider that we have moral duties *to* or *towards* specific subjects. For instance, we seem to owe it *to* another person not to inflict pain on them. The other person is not just a location where we can fulfil a blanket duty not to inflict pain. It is no coincidence that only the affected person can *consent* to having pain inflicted on them, for instance. Neither is it a coincidence that if we have inflicted pain on someone, we must apologise specifically *to them*, and only *they* can forgive us. These are just some of the ways in which the directionality of duties matters.

Kant would affirm all of this. As we have seen in Chap. 2, Kant takes us to have duties *towards* others and duties *towards* self. No duty is directed at no one. Kant furthermore pays close attention to the distinction between a duty *towards* someone and a duty merely *regarding* them (see MM 6:442.01 06). However, despite this eagerness to incorporate directionality into his system of moral philosophy, according to Thompson (2004), Kant has trouble accounting for it on his own terms.

Before explaining the problem in more detail, let me introduce some of the special vocabulary used in this debate. Thompson draws a distinction between 'monadic' and 'bipolar' normative judgements. Monadic normative judgements are judgements such as 'X did wrong in doing A', 'X has a duty to do A', and 'X has a right to do A' (Thompson 2004, 338). These judgements make an explicit reference only to one subject. Contrast this with judgements such as 'X wronged Y by doing A', 'X has a duty to Y to do A', and 'X has a right against Y that he do A' (ibid., 335). These make reference to two subjects and are hence called 'bipolar'.[1] For Thompson, bipolar normative judgements correspond to bipolar normative *relations* or what he calls 'dikaiological orders' under which subjects stand (Thompson 2004, 352). All subjects who can be part of the same bipolar normative relation are called 'persons' relative to that relation (ibid.). For instance, all subjects who can stand in the relation of 'morally owing someone something' are *moral* persons. Similarly, all subjects who can enter into legal relations under Roman law are *legal* persons under the system of Roman law. Finally, the person who bears a duty is called the 'obligor', while the person towards whom the duty is directed is called the 'obligee' (Darwall 2012, 333).

Among other things, it matters how we account for the directionality or 'bipolarity' of moral duties because our account will determine the scope of subjects towards whom these duties can be directed.[2] Thompson's central idea here is that we can only account for bipolarity in terms of *standing under a shared law*. This can be a natural idea if we consider contract law: Two individuals can only enter into a binding contract with each other if they both stand under the same system of contract law.[3] And similarly, if there are to be binding bipolar *moral* relations, it seems they can only obtain between individuals who stand under a shared system of *moral* law. 'Thompson's puzzle', as it is sometimes called, is the challenge to account for the bipolarity of moral duties in terms of a shared moral law

---

[1] Somewhat tendentiously, the word 'bipolar' seems to presuppose that the two subjects referred to in a moral judgement stand on equal footing in some way. Both are 'poles' of the same kind, merely appointed to opposite ends of a moral relation. I am going to deny this mutual equality.

[2] Thompson's own interest in bipolarity rather stems from his interest in *justice*. Justice is understood as a moral virtue agents have, or fail to have, as obligors in bipolar moral relations (Thompson 2004, 337). The just agent does well in fulfilling her moral duties to others, in respecting the moral rights which others have against her, in giving others their moral due, and so on. Moral philosophers who want to account for justice ought therefore to account for bipolar moral relations.

[3] Admittedly, this principle only holds on a fairly authoritarian view of contracts, according to which bindingness derives from some third-party authority. I thank Markus Wild for pointing this out. The bindingness of contracts may simply be a matter of the mutual benefit that results from observance, not of external enforcement. What matters for the present discussion, however, is that the bindingness of Kantian ethical duties depends on a shared moral law just as contracts *on an authoritarian view* depend on a shared legal system.

without dubious assumptions. Thompson claims that Kant, along with Hume and Aristotle, is unable to account for bipolar moral relations in terms of a shared moral law, or at any rate that he would have to rely on "alarming metaphysical commitments" to do so (Thompson 2004, 379). It is helpful to consider this difficulty in more detail because it sheds light on what it means to 'share' the moral law, and why this sharing is so important for interpersonal duties.

Why would Kant fail to account for bipolar moral relations in terms of a shared moral law? Thompson's argument is best illustrated by his own example (Thompson 2004, 361f.): Say the Lombard people have their own system of laws under which all Lombards, and only the Lombards, are legal persons. And say that on the other side of an Alpine mountain range, by sheer coincidence, a people has independently developed which is indistinguishable from the Lombards, down to the language and the legal system. Call these people the Schlombards (though they, of course, call themselves the 'Lombards'). Thompson—convincingly, to my mind—argues that Lombards and Schlombards do not live by *the very same* law, given that their cultures developed in complete isolation from each other. If a Lombard and a Schlombard should happen to meet on the mountain range and attempt to enter into a binding contract with each other, they would fail. They could not enter a binding contract under either Lombard or Schlombard law, since each is not a legal person under the legal system of the other.

The objection to Kant is that his moral philosophy puts moral agents in the position of Lombards and Schlombards (Thompson 2004, 382). For Kant, the moral law is only binding because it is autonomous. It is a self-imposed law. It can only be autonomous, however, because it is also *autochthonous*. That is, it is only a *self-imposed* law because it *originates* in the individual rational being (see Timmermann 2007, 114f.).[4] Therefore, even though all moral agents individually give moral laws to themselves that have *the same content each*, they do not stand under *the very same law*. Their moral laws are distinct in origin and authority. Since they do not stand under the very same moral law, they cannot enter bipolar moral

---

[4] I should add that moral agents give the moral law to themselves *as rational beings*. But considered purely as rational beings, persons have no individual idiosyncrasies—we are not qualitatively different from each other insofar as we are rational beings. However, this does not have to undermine Thompson's point. After all, rational beings are still individuated. We cognise *ourselves* as rational beings. And the bindingness of the moral law for a rational being still hinges on the fact that it is an autonomous law *for that individual rational being*.

relations under that law, argues Thompson. So duties 'towards' other people are impossible for Kant, if Thompson is right. There are only blanket duties, and other people are mere locations where we can fulfil them. Thompson acknowledges that there is one way in which Kant can possibly account for bipolar moral relations. Kant might account for bipolarity by claiming that the moral law does after all have a common origin in all moral agents, namely in pure practical reason, which is not individuated (Thompson 2004, 382). On the one hand, however, this would put a lot of argumentative weight on the claim that pure practical reason is the *singular* or *unified* cause of the moral law, and Thompson takes it that this would be an "alarming metaphysical commitment" (Thompson 2004, 379). Be that as it may, the analogy to Lombards and Schlombards would suggest that in order to be the very same law on Thompson's terms, the moral law would need a common *natural* origin in all moral agents, and it is at least not obvious that a common *nonnatural* origin in pure practical reason will do the trick. It seems, therefore, that Kant indeed faces a difficulty in accounting for bipolarity in terms of a shared moral law.

Kantians have come up with several answers. The most enthusiastic response to Thompson comes from Darwall (2009), who agrees that an autonomous law alone cannot account for bipolar moral relations (Darwall 2009, 138). Accordingly, Darwall advises that a Kantian account of the moral law should start *not* from the notion of an autonomous law alone, but from the notion of second-personal accountability (Darwall 2009, 153). This response to Thompson's challenge obviously comes at a steep price. To agree with Darwall, Kantians would have to sacrifice the view that the moral law is autonomous. But that is to sacrifice an absolutely central element of Kant's moral philosophy.

Fanselow (2008) proposes another response: Moral agents are not merely bound by the moral law in general, but also by *specific duties.* These duties follow from the Categorical Imperative only with the addition of facts about the world. For instance, the duty to hold one's promises derives—on Fanselow's view[5]—from the Formula of Universal Law (FUL) with the addition of certain facts about promising and human psychology (Fanselow 2008, 96). The idea is that the duty not to make false promises follows from the FUL only if we add the fact that in a world of false

---

[5] I do not share Fanselow's suggestion that duties can be *derived* directly from formulations of the Categorical Imperative. As we saw in Chap. 4, Kant rather arrives at specific duties via the doctrine of obligatory ends.

promisers, human beings would not take promises seriously. Since moral agents are all part of the natural world, they share its facts. So even if the moral law is not truly shared among Kantian moral agents, their materially specific duties are based on shared facts. According to Fanselow, this is enough of a shared origin to enable bipolar moral relations at the level of specific duties, and that is what matters.

The main problem with Fanselow's response is that when Thompson asks for a shared origin that accounts for the bindingness of a bipolar moral relation, not just any shared origin will do. By way of analogy, the specific contract into which the Lombard and the Schlombard attempt to enter has a shared natural origin in some respects. The Lombard and the Schlombard have met on the same mountain pass on the same day, have written their contract on the same piece of parchment, and so on. But none of this makes it the case that they indeed stand in a binding legal relation. For that, they would need a common system of contract law. Hence, what would be needed is a common origin of *the system of law under which the contract is binding*, not just a common origin of the contract itself. And since the Lombard and the Schlombard do not stand under the same system of contract law, their contract lacks the right kind of common natural origin. The same holds for Kantian moral agents. Even if they derive their duties from the Categorical Imperative using the same facts, the moral law which makes these duties binding still lacks a common natural origin, and so there is no common normative ground that can account for the bindingness of the Kantian bipolar moral relation. Hence, Fanselow's response is not enough to resolve Thompson's puzzle.

According to another Kantian response (Palatnik 2018), Kantian moral agents usually represent each other as beings with a will. On Palatnik's account, Kantian agents recognise each other in the world of appearances on the basis of "regularities or patterns characteristic of intentional activity" (Palatnik 2018, 294). It thus comes naturally to agents to recognise and represent others as rational beings. Representing others as rational beings however necessarily involves representing them as being bound by the moral law—the *same* moral law under which the agent herself stands (Palatnik 2018, 295). Thus, "we cannot represent (and recognise) anyone as a *practical reasoner*, as *a person in relation to ourselves*, unless we can see him as sharing our basic framework of practical thought, as falling under the principles of pure practical reason and fundamental concepts that follow from these principles" (Palatnik 2018, 300). Therefore, Palatnik's suggestion is that for Kant, a moral agent naturally recognises and represents others as beings bound by the same moral law by which she considers herself to be bound. The claim that Kantian agents can recognise rational—that is, autonomous—beings by natural regularities or patterns might be hard for strict Kantians to accept, but this need not concern us here.[6] What matters is what options are open to Kantians, not whether Kant himself would endorse them. However, Palatnik's suggestion faces a great challenge in solving Thompson's puzzle: It can only account for the bipolar moral relations in which moral agents *take themselves to stand*. It explains why we *consider ourselves to be* bound by bipolar moral relations. But Thompson's puzzle asks for an account of the bipolar relations in which moral agents *actually* stand. For example, the Lombard and the Schlombard represent each other as persons under the same law, but they still fail to enter a binding contract because they do not *actually* stand under the same law. Thus, Palatnik's response is not sufficient to resolve Thompson's puzzle either.

In summary, previous Kantian responses to Thompson's puzzle either face great difficulties, as I argued in the case with Fanselow and Palatnik, or come at a very high cost, as I argued in the case with Darwall. Of course, one could continue the conversation. My point is not that no Kantian solution to Thompson's puzzle is possible. What I hope to have shown, however, is that even the most competent Kantian philosophers have had a surprisingly hard time explaining how a shared moral law is supposed to account for the directionality of Kantian moral duties. This is an area where Kantian ethics stands in dire need of clarification. And this makes it an attractive area for modification.

Consider further that the various responses all strengthen Kant's denial of duties towards animals. On Darwall's account, bipolarity arises from practices or attitudes of holding each other second-personally

---

[6] Kant holds that a being could conceivably have empirical practical reason but not pure practical reason (CPrR 5:449.04–07). These would be beings who can understand and follow hypothetical imperatives, but they would be unable to give themselves the moral law. But of course, such beings would act intentionally. So only because agents can recognise intentional activity, it is not clear that they have to think of others as beings under the moral law. Furthermore, the inference from natural regularities to autonomy would have to be an inference by analogy, as Palatnik acknowledges: "[...] only by *projecting* our own framework of practical thought onto others can we *represent* or *recognise* them as persons at all" (Palatnik 2018, 295). Here, Kant would likely have to disagree. A behaviour that is analogous to rational action, he explicitly emphasises, does not necessarily indicate a rational cause (CPJ 5:464FN). Hence, Kant would not agree that we can recognise other rational beings on the grounds of empirical regularities or patterns.

accountable, in which animals do not participate. On Fanselow's account, bipolarity arises from deriving duties from the Categorical Imperative using facts about the shared natural world, another activity in which animals do not partake. And on Palatnik's account, bipolarity arises from an agent's supposition that the other is bound by the same moral law as herself, which once again is not true for animals. If Kantians want to be able to account for duties towards animals, they should look for a different response to Thompson's puzzle.

It is no coincidence that previous responses to Thompson's puzzle end up excluding animals all the more vehemently. After all, they share with Thompson a crucial assumption: that we must account for bipolar moral relations in terms of a shared moral law. So long as we come up with ways for Kantian ethics to accommodate a shared moral law, the resulting moral philosophy will inevitably exclude animals from moral concern. I therefore suggest a more radical, but also more elegant response to Thompson's puzzle: Kantians should *refuse* to solve it. They should deny altogether that bipolarity, in Thompson's sense of the word, is a feature of the moral landscape. And where there is nothing to be accounted for, there is no puzzle. This is a more robust Kantian response to Thompson, and at the same time it removes a major obstacle for the inclusion of animals in Kantian moral concern.

5.2   First-Personal Versus Second-Personal Accounts of 'Directionality'

To reiterate, Kant himself clearly thinks that only rational beings who mutually share the moral law could have duties 'towards' each other. The underlying reasoning is that only beings who share the moral law can 'necessitate' or 'constrain' each other (MM 6:442.10; see Wood 1998, 189; Korsgaard 2018, 123ff.). It is noteworthy that Kant says the same thing about the juridical domain—animals without legal duties cannot have legal rights because they cannot obligate others, he argues very briefly (MM 6:241.15–17). Thus, the suspicion is not too far-fetched that Kant, like Thompson, draws on an analogy between morality and legal systems when he ties bipolar relations to the sharing of a law. However, I will now suggest that Kant can also inspire a rather different understanding of bipolarity or directionality. This alternative understanding does not rely on the notion of a shared moral law. So we can save Kant with the resources he provides.

To start with, consider some differences between Kant and Thompson when it comes to moral bipolarity. For Thompson, monadic duties form a distinct type from bipolar duties. For instance, according to Thompson there is a monadic duty *not to lie*, over and above the bipolar duty *towards the conversation partner* not to lie (Thompson 2004, 339f.). This corresponds to the intuition that we can feel guilty simply for *having lied*, not only for *having wronged someone by lying* (Thompson 2004, 340). Kant would not draw the distinction in this way. For Kant, *all* duties are bipolar or 'directed' towards an obligating subject, and there is no such thing as a genuinely monadic or 'undirected' duty. Consider the structure of the *Doctrine of Virtue*: Here, Kant makes an exhaustive distinction between duties *to self* and duties *to others* (MM 6:413.07–08). There is no third option. What about Thompson's example of feeling guilty simply for having lied? Kant would agree that a liar has more to feel guilty about than merely having wronged someone else, because we also have a duty *towards self* not to lie (MM 6:429.04–06). But he would flatly deny that there is an 'undirected' duty not to lie.

None of this is to say that Kant is obsessed with the bipolar nature of our duties. He is happy to omit the bipolar element from a duty's description when it is irrelevant. For Kant, the monadic and the bipolar are simply *modes of description*. For Thompson, they are *types of duties*. This is a significant difference. In fact, when Kant and Thompson talk about 'duties towards', they may not be talking about the same thing. And so it is anything but obvious that bipolarity in Thompson's sense must be a feature of the Kantian moral landscape at all. Kant is only committed to bipolarity in his own sense, not Thompson's.

Another, though related difference between Thompson and Kant concerns 'moral authority'. Think of authority as the capacity to create or eradicate duties for someone. Kant's moral philosophy is 'first-personal' in that it derives duties from an autonomous moral law. He considers heteronomy of the will to be "the source of all spurious principles of morality" (G 4:441.02). In Kant's view, then, only the rational being herself has moral authority. Of course, the rational being still has no capacity to create or eradicate duties *at her whim*. Still, duties only derive from the moral law the agent gives to herself. I will call this the 'first-personal Kantian view'. Now, my radical suggestion is that first-personal Kantians should not bother arguing that the moral law is interpersonally 'shared' in any interesting sense. They should stick steadfastly to their claim that the moral law is autonomous and autochthonous, period. And so, for first-personal

Kantians, there is no such thing as second-personal moral authority. Others do not impose the moral law on me, and they consequently cannot create or eradicate any of my duties.

Contrast this view with a 'second-personal Kantianism' along Darwall's lines, which would derive duties from a moral law that is in turn grounded in second-personal accountability (Darwall 2009, 153). The idea is, in a nutshell, that the moral law only arises from acts of second-personal address such as making claims on each other, objecting to each other, holding others answerable, and so on. These acts can, but do not have to, consist in verbal utterances. They can also be reactive attitudes. For instance, we hold others accountable for their wrongdoing simply by *resenting* them. If the moral law derives from such acts of second-personal address, it is an essentially interpersonal law. An important upshot of this is that others have moral authority ('second-personal authority'). They can put others under obligation or lift obligations off their shoulders.[7] For instance, by resenting me, another person puts me under obligation to apologise. By forgiving me, she lifts this obligation off my shoulders.

The view that others have moral authority helps second-personal Kantians account for the bipolarity of duties. We can simply say that duties are directed 'towards' the individual whose moral authority makes it binding.[8] Evidently, this option is not open to first-personal Kantians, who do not believe in this kind of moral authority. How, then, can they account for bipolarity?

Kantians typically insist that "directionality is determined by the source of constraint (your rational will), not by the nature of the resulting object of choice" (Ripstein and Tenenbaum 2020, 147). While this seems like a

[7] Kant evidently has his second-personal moments, for instance, when he asserts that the obligee can always release the obligor (MM 6:417.18–19), or of course in the passages already quoted where he excludes animals as obligees. That is no problem for my point here, because with first-personal Kantianism I merely want to highlight one line of thinking to which Kant's moral philosophy lends itself. My claim is not that Kant unambiguously followed this line of thinking, but only that Kantians could save themselves some trouble by following it.

[8] This is admittedly a truncated version of the second-personal Kantian view. One bit I leave out is the (admittedly important) role of the moral community in second-personal Kantian views. A second-personal Kantian may argue that I have a duty towards X to A if the moral community (of which X is a member) holds me accountable for my doing or omitting A. This however does not change what I am trying to illustrate here, which is that the will of the other—the obligor or the moral community on the obligor's behalf—is involved in giving a duty its normative force on a second-personal Kantian view.

correct representation of Kant's view, it is also a view Kantians can choose to reject. We can go the other way and argue that moral directionality is precisely a matter of what our duties are *about*. According to this view, a duty *towards X* is a duty that is *about X* in a certain way. Never mind who makes a duty binding—consider instead what duties ask us to do and why! Put in Kantian terms, bipolarity is a matter of the *content* or *material* of duty, that is, the end or action we ought to pursue (MM 6:398.5–20). It is not a matter of the *form* of duty, that is, that end or action's character of moral prescription. Call this the *content approach* to bipolarity, as opposed to Thompson's (and Darwall's, Fanselow's, Palatnik's) *form approach.*

How exactly do duties have to be *about X* in order to be duties *towards X*? Interestingly enough, we can gather a version of the content approach from Kant himself. In particular, consider how Kant first introduces the distinction between duties to self and duties to others in the *Doctrine of Virtue* (MM 6:385f.). As we have seen in Chap. 4, Kant here moves from the notion of a Categorical Imperative to that of an 'end that is also a duty' (MM 6:385.31). That is, he moves from the law that prescribes an action unconditionally to the end of that prescribed action. He then draws the central distinction between the obligatory ends insofar as they pertain to our treatment of *others* and *self* (MM 6:385.31–386.14). This is, effectively, how he introduces the two duty-types. And with this conception in mind, we can flesh out the content approach to bipolarity:

The content approach to bipolarity

Any duty is a duty towards self iff it is about the promotion of moral self-perfection.

Any duty is a duty towards another person X iff it is about the promotion of X's happiness.

For the sake of illustration, consider our duties towards self as Kant conceives of them. In particular, take the prohibition of prudential suicide. Our duty not to commit prudential suicide is a duty 'towards self' insofar as it is about our own moral perfection. We ought to keep our natural shape serviceable to morality, and of course being alive is a basic condition for duty-observance (see MM 6:421.10–14). Similarly, our duties towards others are those that are about the promotion of their happiness. Our duty of beneficence is a duty 'towards' others because it is about the promotion of their happiness. Kant's treatment of the end that is also a duty therefore gives us all we need. The content approach to bipolarity suffices to account for the distinction between duties to self and others.

At this point, one might object that the content approach removes Kant's distinction between duties *towards* someone and duties merely *regarding* them. After all, both duties are *about* the same individual. But this objection would miss an important point, namely that the content approach does not equate directionality with 'being-about' in general. For a duty to be a duty *towards X*, it must more specifically be *about X's happiness insofar as it is a part of the obligatory end of the happiness of others*, or *about X's moral perfection insofar as it is a part of the obligatory end of one's own moral perfection*. Duties merely *regarding X* are duties that are about X, but not about X's happiness or moral perfection as part of the obligatory ends.

Consider one of Kant's own examples, the duty not to wantonly destroy beautiful plants (MM 6:443.02–04). This is a duty *regarding* the plant, not *towards* it. This is because the duty is *about the plant*, but *not about the plant's happiness or its moral perfection*. This duty is all about the perfection of the moral agent as part of one of the obligatory ends. Hence, the content approach does not jettison the towards-regarding distinction.

Another objection could be that focusing on content in the proposed way blurs the line between duties towards self and others. One could rightly point out that for Kant, there exists at least one duty that is about our happiness but is a duty towards self: our indirect duty to secure a minimum of happiness for ourselves (G 4:399.03–07; MM 6:388.17–30). But this objection would be flawed too. Consider that this duty is about our own happiness only *insofar as it forms a part of the obligatory end of our own moral perfection*. We should not allow ourselves to become too unhappy, says Kant, because "want of satisfaction with one's condition [...] could easily become a great *temptation to transgression of duty*" (G 4:399.04–07). So even if this duty is about our happiness, it is only about our happiness *as part of the obligatory end of our own moral perfection*. In this way, the content approach upholds the line between duties to self and others.

However, there could be another, more philosophical objection to the content approach to bipolarity. Darwall explicitly argues against the view that duties towards others are just duties with a certain content:

> We can easily imagine a society (Feinberg's 'Nowheresville') in which it is thought morally wrong to step on others' feet, unless, say, they desire or do

not mind one's doing so, but where the latter is not seen as a giving consent that can be understood only within a bipolar dikaiological order. So viewed, others' will and preference would appear simply as features of the moral landscape that bear on moral obligations period. (Darwall 2012, 344f.)

The Nowheresville example illustrates that a duty *towards X* not to step on X's foot is something more than merely a duty *not to step on X's foot*. Rather, according to Darwall's suggestion, duties towards X must be explained in terms of X's second-personal authority, her capacity to obligate the agent under the moral law. By treating others "simply as features of the moral landscape", we turn them into static factors of duty and overlook their subjecthood, or so Darwall worries. Once again, we run the risk of treating others merely as *locations* at which our pursuit of duties can take place (this worry also plagues Korsgaard 2018, 159). In the face of this objection, what can be said on behalf of the content approach?

It is quite intuitive that a duty *towards X* not to step on X's foot is something more specific than merely a duty *not to step on X's foot*. But in itself, that cuts no ice with the content approach. According to this approach, to say that a duty is directed 'towards X' does add something to the duty's description: that it is a duty *about the promotion of X's happiness*. In saying that a duty is directed 'towards X', we indicate that the route of reasoning to this duty passes through the obligatory end of others' happiness. So the first-personal Kantian simply agrees with Darwall that the bipolar element adds something to a duty's description. But it adds nothing that needs accounting for in second-personal terms.

What about Darwall's more general worry that morality without second-personal elements leads to 'Nowheresville'? Are others bound to be mere 'features of the moral landscape' on a first-personal view? Yes and no. First-personal Kantians deny that others can help *bring about* the moral landscape. The moral landscape exists because—and *only* because—the moral agent gives the moral law to herself. In this sense, others really are just features of the moral landscape. They register on a radar set up by rational beings from the first-person standpoint. But this does not imply that others cannot play a unique role in determining what actions are prescribed. Recall that for Kant, "what [others] may count as belonging to their happiness is left to their own judgement" (MM 6:388.08–09). The more we emphasise the role of another's agency as a guide for our practical benevolence, the more active their involvement in our duties is. Therefore, we should not conceive of others as *static* features of the moral landscape. They are uniquely *dynamic* features. The first-personal Kantian view is sensitive to the fact that others are active subjects. What is denied is only that the subjecthood of others helps to *create* or *eradicate* any parts of the moral landscape.

5.3   Rejecting Thompson's Challenge

Against this backdrop of Kantian conceptions, let me propose a novel response to Thompson's puzzle. To reiterate, the puzzle is the challenge of accounting for moral bipolarity in terms of a shared moral law. Kantians have trouble meeting this challenge. I have now argued that Kant's view of bipolarity differs from Thompson. In fact, the words 'duty towards X' may mean something quite different for the two.

First-personal Kantians cannot account for bipolarity in terms of a shared moral law. We must accept this. But that is not to admit defeat in the face of Thompson's puzzle, to the contrary! Rather, first-personal Kantians can simply deny that bipolarity in Thompson's sense exists. Our duties simply do not have any feature that needs accounting for in second-personal terms. To be sure, this is not a solution to Thompson's puzzle, but a rejection of its presupposition. This rejection also avoids the difficulties of previous responses to the puzzle: controversial metaphysical commitments (Thompson's Kant), the Lombard-Schlombard problem (Fanselow, Palatnik), and the exclusion of animals from direct moral consideration (all of the above, also Darwall).

It may seem that what I propose is easier said than done. After all, the conception of bipolarity we find in Thompson and Darwall is supposed to describe certain aspects of moral life. Moral life, the basic idea goes, consists not just of monadic duties. It consists of essentially *interpersonal* relations. We owe things to each other, object to each other, forgive each other, and so on. To use Thompson's term, the moral landscape is full of 'dikaiological orders'.

For second-personal Kantians, interpersonal relations uniquely connect obligor and obligee.[9] Part of this is that the obligee has a special standing vis à vis the obligor. Case in point: Only obligees have the power to *consent* (Darwall 2012, 345). And when they have been wronged, obligees have a

---

[9] To repeat, the obligee is the subject towards whom there exists a duty. The obligor is the subject who has the duty (Darwall 2012, 333).

special standing too: Only the obligee can *forgive* the wrongdoer, and only the obligee is owed *apologies* (Darwall 2012, 346). Naturally, Darwall would explain these features of moral life under reference to second-personal authority (Darwall 2012, 347). As first-personal Kantians who follow the content approach, are we to flatly deny that moral life has these features? Is everybody in a position to consent for anyone else? Can everybody forgive wrongdoers? Do wrongdoers have to apologise to everybody equally?

Fortunately, no such absurd claims follow. First-personal Kantians can account for ordinary practices of consenting, forgiving, and apologising, with different means. They can use what I will call the 'deflate-and-deny tactic':

The deflate-and-deny tactic

For any supposed exercise of second-personal authority, deflate it, as far as possible, to an exercise of the moral authority of the moral agent plus the capacity of others to determine the content of an agent's duty. Deny the rest.

To give a preliminary example: Consider the ordinary practice of forgiving others for past wrongs. Darwall would consider forgiveness to be an act of release-from-duty. Among other things, to forgive someone is to release them from the duty to make amends. But we do not have the power to release others from any of their duties on a first-personal Kantian view. Either they have a duty to make amends that derives from the autonomously imposed moral law, or they do not. Us others have no say in the matter. What the first-personal Kantian can say, however, is that to verbally forgive is to provide information about the conditions of one's happiness. Broadly, it is to signal that one is 'over it'. The obligee verbally forgives the wrongdoer and thus makes it clear that no more amends are required for her happiness. This does not change anything about the wrongdoer's duties, but it makes it clear that making further amends are not what their duties towards the obligee demand of them. This is the 'deflate' bit of the tactic. What the first-personal Kantian cannot account for is forgiveness as an act of literally lifting a duty off the obligor's shoulders, and so she should simply deny that this is possible. We have no power to create or eliminate the duties of others. This is the 'deny' bit of the tactic.

Deflate-and-deny is a *tactic* because it can be applied in various contexts. No matter which specific examples adherents of second-personal authority bring up, deflate-and-deny can be applied. Of course, the tactic must prove its worth in particular applications, but it would be futile to attempt a comprehensive list of supposedly 'second-personal' aspects of moral life.[10] To second-personal Kantians, the moral landscape is saturated with second-personal authority. In Sect. 5.4, let me merely attempt to illustrate the proposed tactic by discussing Darwall's most prominent, aforementioned examples: consent, forgiveness, and apologies. We will see that so much about the giving and obtaining of consent, about forgiving, and about apologising can be 'deflated'—particularly to the determining of the content of another's duties and informing them about it—that very little has to be 'denied'. The first-personal Kantian thus does not have to reject these moral practices, just their explanation in second-personal terms.

5.4   CONSENT, FORGIVENESS, AND APOLOGIES WITHOUT SECOND-PERSONAL AUTHORITY

Darwall makes it clear that he conceives of giving consent as "an exercise of a 'normative power', in this case, to release someone from a bipolar obligation he would otherwise have" (Darwall 2012, 345). Consent is thus, like forgiveness, an instance of release-from-duty. As we have already seen, we have no such power to create or eradicate duties for others on a first-personal Kantian view. Therefore, the deflate-and-deny tactic should be applied to release-from-duty, and by extension to consent.

A part of what Darwall means by 'releasing' someone from their duty can be deflated to powers the first-personal Kantian can accept: (1) We can *inform* others that what they think is their duty is not in fact their duty. For example, I can inform others that I have no desire to drink coffee, implying that their duty towards me to promote my happiness in no way requires that they buy me coffee; (2) We can *set ends*, or *reorder* our ends. Since others should promote our happiness primarily by assisting us in our

---

[10] Some more examples that come to mind are promising (Darwall 2006, 203ff.) demanding something (Schaber 2014), morally blaming others, complaining or objecting to others, or prohibiting others from doing things. The deflate-and-deny tactic is meant to apply to all of these examples. Of course, it would take much more work to defend the results of the deflate-and-deny tactic on philosophical grounds—to show that purely first-personal accounts of supposedly second-personal practices can be adequate. I do not claim to do that work here. My aim is merely to sketch the general direction in which Kantianism for Animals would take us.

own endeavours, this changes what others should do. For example, if I initially had the desire to have coffee, but noticed that I did not bring any money and would have to rely on a favour from a colleague, I might reconsider whether I really want any coffee given the circumstances. In both situations, it would be perfectly reasonable for me to tell my colleague "it's alright, you don't have to buy me coffee". With my utterance I would not have lifted any duty from my colleague's shoulders. My colleague's duty is still what it was, namely to promote my happiness. But by signalling the conditions of my happiness, I would have provided a clue regarding the content of the other person's duty. That is enough.

What the first-personal Kantian cannot account for, of course, is the supposed act of literally *erasing* someone else's duty. Here, the 'deny' part of the deflate-and-deny tactic comes into play: The first-personal Kantian simply denies that this act is possible. If the obligee really has a duty towards us, it is not in our power to erase it. This has implications for the limits of our power to 'release' others from their duties: We can give false or misleading information about what another's duty is (say, out of politeness). Others should not take such utterances at face value. For example, suppose I politely tell my colleague "it's okay, you don't have to buy me coffee", but really I would love to have a cup. In this case, my colleague's duty to promote my happiness still demands buying me coffee. What matters is not any internal or external act of second-personal address, but my happiness.[11]

Put in this way, the first-personal Kantian view is likely much stricter than Kant's own view. Kant evidently thinks that if X has a duty towards Y, then Y can always release X from that duty at will. This is the assumption that raises the basic problem with duties to self in the *Doctrine of Virtue* (MM 6:417.07–22). The problem is this: It would seem, at first sight, that duties towards self could not be stable, because we could release ourselves from these duties at will (ibid.). Evidently, this problem only arises if we understand release-from-duty as a literal *erasure* of duty by an act of the

---

[11] Conversely, we cannot erase our own moral *rights* on the first-personal Kantian view I propose. On an orthodox Kantian view, rights are grounded in duties, not vice versa. We have rights against others simply in the sense that they have certain duties against us. Therefore, if we cannot erase another's duties, we cannot erase our rights. However, this does not make our rights static. After all, which duties others have against us is contingent on what promotes our happiness, which we in turn shape by setting happiness-derived ends. In one sense, then, all rights are inalienable on the first-personal Kantian view, but in another sense they can be acquired and lost as a consequence of acts of instrumental practical reason.

obligee's will. Kant's solution is that duties to self are really duties of the *homo phaenomenon*—the human being as a subject of inclinations—to the *homo noumenon*—the human being as a subject of a rational will (MM 6:418.14–23). But it is not as though Kant really struggled with this problem. Rather, posing and resolving the problem serves a heuristic function. Kant's discussion illuminates the nature of duties to self: When we owe something to 'ourselves', we owe it to ourselves purely as rational beings. Kant could have made the same point without using this specific problem as a heuristic device. What is more, the underlying assumption that obligees can eradicate duties at will does not seem to carry any weight anywhere else in Kant's oeuvre. Kant does not mention it in other contexts, let alone build any elaborate arguments upon it. So Kantians can confidently dispense with the assumption that obligees can eradicate duties at will. No serious difficulties follow.

What happens if we apply the first-personal view of release-from-duty to the more specific case of giving consent? On Darwall's conception, if Y consents to X's doing A, then Y releases X from the duty towards Y not to do A (Darwall 2012, 345). For instance, a patient may consent to a surgical procedure, thus releasing the medical personnel from the duty to refrain from that procedure, say, out of respect for bodily integrity. Darwall emphasises that by giving consent, we do more than merely to inform another that we "do not mind" (Darwall 2012, 344). On the first-personal Kantian view, however, it is just that. Or at any rate, to give consent is *either* to inform others about their duty *or* to make up one's mind so that it becomes clear what their duty is. In certain circumstances, this may indeed amount to no more than saying that one does not mind. For instance, if a medical patient has her priorities in clear order and knows the impact of a procedure on her happiness, she can inform the medical personnel that their duty to promote her happiness does not require that they refrain from this procedure. In other cases, however, the story may be much more complicated. Perhaps the patient does not initially have a clear picture of whether she prefers the consequences of the procedure to the consequences of its omission. In such cases, obtaining the patient's consent also forces her to make up her mind. In either case, the patient is not *eradicating* any duties on the part of the medical personnel, but merely makes it clearer what the content of their duties is.

The first-personal view on giving consent may invite the worry that it confers the power to consent on too many people. It seems to confer this power on anyone who can provide good information about that person's happiness. But it does not. First, the patient's happiness may depend on the very right to determine *herself* whether she allows the procedure. Human beings usually do not like being paternalised, and our practical benevolence should be sensitive to this fact.[12] Secondly, the patient of course has better epistemic access to the conditions of her own happiness and to the ends by means of which she aims to achieve it. In typical cases, patients will therefore be in a uniquely privileged position to give consent to actions which impact them. And this unique position should be our reference point when we conceive of the position in which one should be to validly give consent at all. On this conception, usually only the impacted subject will be in a position to consent.

However, exceptions are possible. There might be *uninformed* or *misinformed* obligees, and the first-personal Kantian can easily explain why we should not take their consent at face value. They are, at least in this instance, not good enough informants about the conditions of their own happiness. There could also be *irrational* patients: They know the ends whose realisation would make them happy, and they know the procedure is not conducive to these ends, yet they fail to rationally combine these pieces of information. Even though withholding consent would be in their best interest, they consent. Suppose there are others who have, let us assume, heard a comprehensive and true firsthand account of the patient's desires and ends, and of the procedure's harmful impact. On a first-personal Kantian view, those rational and informed others may be in a better position to give or deny consent than the patient. The crucial and difficult question is, of course, who is to count as uninformed, misinformed, or irrational. It merits philosophical attention in its own right. What is clear from a Kantian point of view, however, is that arrogance is a vice, and self-serving rationalisations are a straightforward danger. So we should approach the question whose consent counts with humility, even though we do not get to simply avoid it. We must not simply presume that we know better what is good for others than they themselves do.

So far, the first-personal Kantian take on consent may sound largely destructive. But there are also more constructive upshots, particularly

---

[12] This is not always the case. There may be decisions about which people do not care, and regarding which they have no special intent of making a decision for themselves. For the first-personal Kantian, such indifferent consent does not carry much weight, nor does the omission of indifferent consent. After all, it gives us, the obligors, no useful information about the happiness of the obligee.

when we think about consent as it applies to animals: For traditional, second-personal Kantians, the fact that animals cannot consent makes a world of difference.[13] It indicates that animals cannot have moral authority, do neither put us under obligation nor lift duties off our shoulders, and more generally are not proper objects of moral concern in their own right. Not so on the first-personal view. Here, the obtaining and giving of consent is merely a means of conveying information about desires, practical ends, and their ordering, or to make up our minds. What really matters at the end of the day is not an act of second-personal address. What matters is that the obligor gets the conditions of the obligee's happiness right. Animals do not speak a human language. Still, we can take steps to get it right what makes them happy (for instance, paying close attention, counteracting our own biases, considering scientific evidence). The fact that animals cannot consent, be it verbally or by reactive attitude, is of little consequence. It merely shows that we should take alternative measures to ensure that we get the conditions of an animal's happiness right, given that they cannot verbally tell us what our duty demands. Paying close attention to the animal and relying on the best information we have about its well-being can serve largely the same purpose as the obtaining of informed consent from human beings. It should be treated as equally morally important.

A similar difference emerges when we compare Darwall and the first-personal Kantian on the topic of forgiveness. On Darwall's view, "forgiveness acknowledges the other's responsibility for wronging one, but refrains from pressing claims or 'holding it against' him" (Darwall 2009, 72). By 'pressing claims' and 'holding it against him', Darwall means the exercise of second-personal moral authority. To 'press claims' is, among other things,[14] to create or keep in existence a duty for the wrongdoer to apologise, to blame herself, or to make amends for her wrongdoing. Darwall's

---

[13]What makes the difference is not that animals *do not* consent, but that they *cannot*. Darwall emphasises that second personal authority is not entirely a matter of *actual* acts of second-personal address on behalf of the obligee (Darwall 2007, 64). Rather, it is a matter of acts of second-personal address which the obligee—or indeed the moral community of which she is a part—is *prone* to make (ibid.). However, none of this changes the fact that it is acts of second-personal address of some kind that create or eradicate duties on Darwall's view. This is what the first-personal Kantian should deny.

[14]Darwall himself mainly emphasises the role of *reactive attitudes*, particularly of resentment (see Darwall 2012, 346). To 'press claims' is to take a resentful attitude towards an obligee. That however not the bit of the story with which the first-personal Kantian must disagree, and for this reason I leave it aside.

picture is that wronging someone leads to special duties of the wrongdoer to the wronged, and thus the wronged are obligees with a special authority to free the wrongdoer from these special duties (see Darwall 2012, 356).

We can account for part of what Darwall means by 'forgiveness' in first-personal Kantian terms: A verbal utterance of forgiveness can serve the purpose of informing someone that apologising, self-blame, or amends are not the content of her duty. For instance, X may forgive Y for having stolen an inconsequential amount of money several years ago. In the end, no harm came to X from Y's theft, and the utterance of forgiveness is quite simply a way of communicating this fact. In verbally forgiving Y, X signals that the promotion of her happiness does not require reparations for this act. Perhaps in this example, verbal forgiving may be a somewhat vacuous ritual. But in other cases, verbal forgiving can convey crucial information about a person's happiness. Say X neglected the infant Y, who has now grown up. The adult Y's utterance of forgiveness for X may convey the—anything but obvious!—information that Y's happiness is no longer impacted by this serious wrong. And even much more complicated arrangements are conceivable. For instance, forgiving may be an intrapersonal process through which someone who has been wronged actively *emancipates* herself from the impact of past wrongdoing. In forgiving, one performatively denies the wrongdoer any lasting impact. In this case, verbal forgiving is not merely an *informative* act, but also an act of self-assertion.

On the other hand, the first-personal Kantian cannot agree with everything that Darwall says about forgiveness. For a first-personal Kantian, forgiving others cannot be an act of lifting any duties off their shoulders. Just as the first-personal Kantian view limits our power to consent, it limits our power to forgive. Our utterances of forgiveness, like our utterances of consent, can convey false or misleading information, and in these instances we should not take them at face value (except perhaps as performative self-assertions).

When it comes to animals, the implications of the first-personal Kantian view on forgiveness echo what I have said about consent. Animals do not forgive, but on its own this is of little consequence. What matters is that we get the conditions of another's happiness right, because that is what we must promote. And of course, the conditions of an animal's happiness can be shaped by our past wrongs, and animals can 'get over' that influence over time. Animals who have suffered a certain type of abuse may have different needs than their conspecifics who have not. Our duties are sensitive to such individual differences in happiness. Hence, it is crucial that we pay close attention to how our actions have impacted an animal and how we can promote its happiness specifically against the backdrop of our wrongs.

Apologies are, among other things, pleas for forgiveness. Darwall conceives of apologies partly as pleas for the eradication of special duties that wronging someone creates, perhaps a duty to blame oneself or a duty to make reparations.[15] One quite intuitive upshot of this conception is that apologies must be directed only *from the wrongdoer to the wronged* (Darwall 2012, 346). Nobody else can apologise for this particular wrong, and one can apologise to nobody but the wronged. After all, Darwall's view entails that only the wronged has the authority of an obligee to free the obligor from her duties (ibid.).

Again, the first-personal Kantian can deflate part of what Darwall means by 'apologies'. The first hint comes from Darwall himself: "If a victim comes upon an unaddressed admission of guilt and expression of sincere regret in her victimiser's diary, she has not discovered an apology" (ibid.). Of course, it is true that the verbal *expression of apology* must always be addressed to the wronged. But it is a separate question whether the *duty to apologise* is always owed to the person to whom the verbal utterance is addressed.

For Darwall, apologies are crucially *more* than admissions of guilt and regret. For the first-personal Kantian, they are basically that, plus perhaps an expression of *resolve* to act better in the future. To issue such utterances may be our duty to others. After all, it is quite plausible that apologies promote the happiness of those we have wronged. For instance, apologies often lead to forgiveness, and forgiveness is good for our mental health and well-being (see Toussaint and Webb 2005). So apologies can be a formidable way for wrongdoers to promote the happiness of the wronged, in a way no one else can. But apologies may also give the person we have wronged some pleasant reassurance that, having acknowledged the wrongness of their action, the wrongdoer is less likely to repeat it. The first-personal Kantian therefore has some foothold to argue that apologies are owed to the obligee based on the duty to promote their happiness. This also explains why a secret expression of guilt in a diary cannot serve the usual purpose of an apology, since it is not intended to promote the

---

[15] Again, this is not the part of Darwall's conception that he emphasises most, but it is the part with which the first-personal Kantian must take issue.

happiness of the wronged. It is equally clear, however, that exceptions are possible such that apologies do not promote the happiness of those we have wronged. For instance, if the wrong in question is very grave, an apology may indeed trivialise it. Sometimes, 'sorry' does not cut it. In such cases, it would indeed go *against* our duty towards others to apologise.

However, we may still have a duty towards *self* to apologise to those we have wronged. Our duties to self, on the first-personal Kantian conception, are about moral self-perfection. Apologies serve this end by helping us cultivate a sense of duty. The practice of apologising forces us to recall our wrongs and to indulge in feelings of guilt. If we additionally conceive of apologies as expressions of resolve to act better in the future, it is even more evident how this ritual promotes moral self-perfection. Apologies help us act better next time around.

The first-personal Kantian still denies that apologies should be understood as pleas to be freed from the special duties we incur by wronging others, since that plea would be impossible for others to fulfil. Obligees cannot eradicate our duties. Yet again, the focus is shifted away from the act of second-personal address and onto the purpose it serves. The apologies we ought to utter, in one way or another, serve to promote the happiness of others or our own moral perfection. What matters is that we achieve these obligatory ends rather than that we use the specific means of a verbal act of second-personal address.

Again, there are constructive upshots regarding animals. Like consent and forgiveness, apologies are means to an end. But there may be other, much more important ways to achieve that same end. This is so even with apologies when it comes to animals. Animals cannot understand apologies. Instead, we can take extra care in determining how to promote an animal's happiness in the special context of our past wrongs. When I have stepped on a cat's tail, I can pay special attention to whether any lasting injury has come from my wrong.

However, since we also have a duty to *self* to apologise, as a sort of moral exercise, it may even be our duty to issue a verbal apology to animals. As silly as it may sound at first, apologising to animals is already a common practice. Imagine a person who trips over a black cat in the dark and feels guilty for not having been more careful. It would be a perfectly understandable and reasonable reaction to exclaim "oh no, I'm sorry!" and then check if the cat is hurt and attempt to comfort her. The former is a verbal apology addressed to the animal and the latter is an alternative measure to make up for the wrong in terms of the happiness of the animal.

On a first-personal Kantian view, our practice of apologising to animals is not just an irrational spillover effect from our moral interactions with humans. It can be a perfectly fine example of the fulfilment of a duty to self to apologise, based on the duty of moral self-perfection.

Let me sum up. In this chapter I have addressed a major difficulty for Kantians in including animals as moral patients: As Kant sees it, we can only have duties towards beings who share our moral law. This is because, in the view of Kant and many Kantians, our duties only have their bipolar or 'directed' character due to our sharing of the moral law. This view however stands in tension with the fact that, on a traditional Kantian view, the moral law is autonomous and autochthonous. It is not in any straightforward sense 'shared'. In response, Kantians typically try to explain how the moral law is after all shared between Kantian agents. I have suggested the opposite move: Kantians should double down on the commitment that the moral law is *not* shared in any ambitious sense, but rather arises from the individual rational being alone. Instead of trying to account for moral bipolarity in terms of a shared moral law, we should account for it in terms of the *content* of our duties. Duties *towards* X are duties that are *about* X in a certain way. I have spelled out this 'content approach' for duties of virtue: Duties to self are about moral self-perfection, and duties to others are about others' happiness.

Some would object that this approach is blind to an essential part of moral life, namely the part that involves second-personal authority. How could this approach explain, say, an obligee's unique standing to give consent, to forgive a wrongdoer, or to demand apologies? Do we not need to appeal to the obligee's capacity to put us under obligation and free us from obligation? To deal with such examples, I employ the 'deflate-and-deny tactic': Deflate any given part of moral life to something for which you can account in terms of first-personal Kantianism, and boldly deny the rest. I have illustrated the tactic on the three examples of consent, forgiveness, and apologies.

I hope to have shown in this chapter what first personal Kantianism is, and that it can bring us a crucial step closer to including animals in Kantian moral concern. What remains to be done now is to see how much of Kant's framework we can actually 'translate' onto our treatment of animals if we take the steps proposed so far. That is the task of the next chapter.

References

Darwall, Stephen. 2006. *The second-person standpoint: Morality, respect, and accountability.* Cambridge, MA: Harvard University Press.

Darwall, Stephen. 2007. Reply to Korsgaard, Wallace, and Watson. *Ethics* 118: 52–69.

Darwall, Stephen. 2009. Why Kant needs the second-person standpoint. In *The Blackwell guide to Kant's ethics*, ed. Thomas E. Hill, 138–158. Malden, MA: Wiley-Blackwell.

Darwall, Stephen. 2012. Bipolar obligation. In *Oxford studies in metaethics vol. 7*, ed. Russ Shafer-Landau, 333–357. Oxford: Oxford University Press.

Fanselow, Ryan. 2008. A Kantian solution to Thompson's puzzle about justice. *Proceedings of the XXII World Congress of Philosophy* 10: 91–99.

Korsgaard, Christine M. 2018. *Fellow creatures: Our obligations to the other animals.* Oxford: Oxford University Press.

Palatnik, Nataliya. 2018. Kantian agents and their significant others. *Kantian Review* 23: 285–306.

Ripstein, Arthur, and Sergio Tenenbaum. 2020. Directionality and virtuous ends. In *Kant and animals*, ed. John J. Callanan and Lucy Allais, 139–156. Oxford: Oxford University Press.

Schaber, Peter. 2014. Demanding something. *Grazer Philosophische Studien* 90: 63–77.

Sensen, Oliver. 2011. *Kant on human dignity.* Berlin: De Gruyter.

Thompson, Michael. 2004. What is it to wrong someone? A puzzle about justice. In *Reason and value: Themes from the moral philosophy of Joseph Raz*, ed. R. Jay Wallace, Philip Pettit, Samuel Scheffler, and Michael Smith, 333–384. Oxford: Oxford University Press.

Timmermann, Jens. 2007. *Kant's Groundwork of the Metaphysics of Morals: A commentary.* Cambridge: Cambridge University Press.

Timmermann, Jens. 2014. Kant and the second-person standpoint. *Grazer Philosophische Studien* 90: 131–147.

Toussaint, Loren, and Jon R. Webb. 2005. Theoretical and empirical connections between forgiveness, mental health and well-being. In *Handbook of forgiveness*, ed. Everett L. Worthington, 349–362. New York: Routledge.

Wood, Allen W. 1998. Kant on duties regarding non-rational nature. *Aristotelian Society Supplementary Volume 72*: 189–210.

CHAPTER 6

Kantian Moral Patients Without Practical Reason?

6.1 Duties of Respect Towards Moral Non-Agents?

So far, I have suggested a way to understand the Categorical Imperative so that animals are not inherently excluded from moral concern (Chap. 4), and I have proposed an alternative to Kant's view of directionality, according to which there can be duties towards animals (Chap. 5). It would be convenient if we could now simply apply Kant's taxonomy of duties from the *Doctrine of Virtue* to the domain of animals as moral patients. We would effectively have transformed Kant's oeuvre on ethics into an oeuvre on animal ethics. Unfortunately, Kant's tacit (and sometimes not-so-tacit) assumption that all moral patients are finite rational beings leads to two additional difficulties. First, Kant assumes that all moral agents and patients are subjects of pure practical reason, who are equal in moral potential. This gives rise to a special class of duties—duties of respect—which demand that we do not exalt ourselves above others (MM 6:449.32). More specifically, duties of respect rule out not only being arrogant or contemptuous towards others, but also being overbearingly beneficent. Thus, duties of respect put a crucial limit on beneficence and put an important qualifier to the demands of duties of love. This gives rise to the characteristically Kantian idea that we should seek the right *balance* or *reconciliation* between beneficence and non-exaltation.

Secondly, as we saw in Chap. 2, Kant's conception of practical love revolves around the idea that others pursue their own happiness as a

N. D. Müller, *Kantianism for Animals*, The Palgrave Macmillan Animal Ethics Series, https://doi.org/10.1007/978-3-031-01930-2_6

matter of instrumental rationality. Because others set their ends with an eye to happiness, our best way of promoting their happiness is to support their self-chosen ends. But animals, at least as Kant sees them, are incapable of consciously pursuing their happiness as an end. Indeed, they pursue no 'ends' at all, being entirely steered by blind instinct (CPJ 5:172.10). Thus, Kant's discussion of duties towards others rests on the assumption that others are subjects of both *pure practical reason* and *instrumental practical reason*. In this chapter, I will argue that with some modifications to the taxonomy, we can accommodate the ideas of duties of respect and of love even towards animals. Considering these duties in more detail also helps to see what our duties towards animals demand according to Kantianism for Animals.

Let me begin with the first difficulty, which concerns duties of respect. As we have already seen in Chap. 2, Kant describes these duties as a force of "repulsion" (MM 6:470.05), in that they ask us not to encroach upon others. They act as an important counterweight to duties of love, which on their own would simply demand that we benefit others without any limit. The reason why we ought not to encroach upon others is that, in doing so, we would be 'exalting' ourselves above them (see MM 6:449.32). In Kant's view, generosity burdens the beneficiary with the expectation of politeness and flattery (*Collins* 27:341f.), putting her on an unequal footing with the benefactor. The very existence of duties of respect is thus predicated, first, on the assumption of moral equality, and secondly on moral agency and social expectations. But none of this appears to apply to animals, who are neither moral agents nor our moral equals.

As mentioned in Chap. 2, duties of respect present a taxonomical puzzle (Fahmy 2013). Kant categorises them as duties towards others, yet they do not appear to derive from the obligatory end of the happiness of others. Indeed, an important point about these duties is that they *limit* the extent to which we should be beneficent towards others. Kant also categorises duties of respect as duties of virtue, yet they do not appear to prescribe an end we should adopt, only the negative condition (MM 6.449.32, Baron 2002, 399) that we should not exalt ourselves above others in various ways. Whatever the solution to this taxonomical puzzle is, Kant clearly takes the recognition of another's humanity—more importantly, their *equal* humanity!—to give rise to a duty not to exalt ourselves above them.

At first sight, it is hard to see how something like a Kantian duty of respect towards others could be justified along the lines of Kantianism for Animals. In this framework, a duty *counts* as a duty 'towards' others if, and only if, it derives from the obligatory end of the happiness of others (see Sect. 5.2 above). Of course, Kantianism for Animals can ask that we do not go so blatantly overboard in our attempts at beneficence that they backfire and make others less happy. But this is less a counterweight to the demands of duties of love than a built-in restriction of beneficence itself. What is more, animals are not our moral equals. They do not stand under a moral law, and they do not share our moral predicament. There simply seems to be no equality to be acknowledged here. So how could there arise a duty to acknowledge equality and not exalt ourselves above them? Do we have to abandon entirely the idea of a reconciliation of love and non-exaltation, of beneficence and recognition of equality?

The answer, I want to suggest, is no. We can preserve a part of the idea that we should not exalt ourselves above others even if those others are animals. We can even preserve the idea that this duty of non-exaltation is connected to the recognition of something like equality. But we need to depart from Kant one more time in order to do so in a way that considers animals. The first step to the solution is to put the duty of non-exaltation in another part of Kant's taxonomy. In Kantianism for Animals, we should understand this duty not as a duty *towards others*, but as a duty *to self, merely regarding others*.[1] This represents another departure from Kant (though one concerning a point on which, as we have seen, his taxonomy stands in need of clarification anyway). Of course, this move is not without a certain irony, given that Kant made the same move the other way around, declaring our most important duties regarding animals to be duties to self. Conversely, in Kantianism for Animals, it is precisely those duties that would appear to hold only towards human beings, in virtue of their equal humanity, that are truly duties to self. If they still appear like duties towards others, that is an amphiboly in moral concepts of reflection.

Duties to self, on the conception outlined in Chap. 5, are those which derive from the obligatory end of our own moral perfection. This 'perfection' consists, on the one hand, in keeping ourselves in good moral shape as duty-observers (e.g. by not increasing our inclinations by overindulging in food, drugs, or sexuality, MM 6:427.01–428.26; MM 6:424.09–425.36).

---

[1] There is an exception to this claim, namely the duty to benefit others' qualitatively moral happiness. As we saw in Sect. 2.3, Kant acknowledges that there are qualitatively moral sensations, such as pangs of conscience or being morally content with oneself. Not to create such qualitatively moral pains in other human beings can be conceived as a duty directly towards others even according to Kantianism for Animals.

On the other hand, it consists in recognising, and acting in accordance with, proper moral self-esteem. We should not lower ourselves below others with whom we are truly "on a footing of equality" (MM 6:434.04), for instance by being servile (MM 6:434.20–436.13). But it seems perfectly plausible that the end of moral perfection, so understood, also requires that we do not exalt ourselves *above* our equals. In being arrogant, we "expect other human beings to esteem themselves but little in comparison with us" (MM 6:465.12–13). This expectation, just like the converse expectation that others should *not* respect us as potential observers of the moral law, is not appropriate to our equal status as moral agents. So the duty of non-exaltation fits the description of a duty to self in Kant's framework very straightforwardly.

Recategorising the duty of non-exaltation as a duty to self makes sense on another count too: It emphasises how this duty is truly about a form of humility concerning ourselves, as much as it is about other-regarding stances. The duties Kant lists as specifications—not to be arrogant, not to backbite, not to ridicule others—are fundamentally about the recognition of a *relation* between equals. Another upside of the recategorisation I advocate is that the duty of non-exaltation can still play the role of a counterweight or limiting condition to the demands of duties of love, since in general duties to self and duties to others must be reconciled (see Vogt 2009, 238).

However, it must be said that conceiving of duties of respect as duties to self also presents some apparent problems. First, ordinary moral experience would suggest that we owe it *to others* not to be arrogant towards them or exalt ourselves above them in other ways. Is it not strange to claim that we truly only wrong ourselves by being arrogant? Consider, however, that Kantianism for Animals does not have to claim that *acting* from arrogance in a way that harms others only wrongs ourselves. As soon as the happiness of others is affected, our duties to others give us a foothold for moral criticism. What is at issue here is the duty we violate merely by having an *supposition* that others should view themselves as below us, the *inner* exaltation by which we see ourselves as inherently more worthy than others. That this type of exaltation should violate only a duty to self does not seem so strange.

Secondly, there is the further problem that Kant views only duties of respect as *owed* duties, while duties of love are *meritorious* (see Chap. 2). If we recategorise duties of respect as duties to self, only meritorious duties to others remain. Does that mean that we never owe others anything? This would again appear to conflict with ordinary moral experience, where we do seem to owe a certain treatment to others (including animals). However, recall that when Kant calls a duty 'meritorious', he does not mean to say it is not a duty. Others can morally object to our failure to observe meritorious duties, and those most affected by our failings are often in the best position to point them out. So, importantly, the meritorious is not the supererogatory. Kant draws the owed-meritorious distinction mainly by appeal to whether observance of a duty puts the other under a reciprocal obligation (say, to be grateful). But we should not expect this to be a very important distinction in an ethical system designed to capture duties towards animals, who can never acquire obligations anyway.

When it comes to capturing the ordinary experience of feeling like we 'owe' another some treatment, we are better served by a perfect-imperfect distinction than Kant's owed-meritorious distinction. This perfect-imperfect distinction applies to our duties of love towards others as much as to our duties to self. What we 'owe' others is what anyone could expect us to do, a duty which we can have no good reason *not* to observe. That is a feature characteristic of perfect duties, which we can observe in every single instance. Imperfect duties, by contrast, are those that require a choice concerning when and how to observe them. Although anyone could expect us to observe our imperfect duties at some point in some way, there can be good reasons in terms of other (perfect or imperfect) duties that keep us from observing them in any particular instance. Now, since duties of virtue according to Kant prescribe the adoption of a certain end, they are always 'wide' and can get in each other's way. However, to every duty of virtue there correspond 'vices'—stances such as arrogance or contempt, which run counter to the observance of our duties. While the positive duty to adopt a certain end is never truly perfect, the duty *not* to adopt and act on a contravening vice is perfect. Even if we cannot always, without restriction, adopt an end of beneficence or sympathetic participation, we *can* always *not* take pleasure in another's misfortune. To capture the feeling of owing others something, we should appeal to such a perfect-imperfect distinction as it applies to our duties of love and their corresponding vices.

Assuming that what Kant calls 'duties of respect' can be recategorised as duties to self, there remains the problem that these duties hinge on the recognition of moral equality. The reason why we should not go overboard in our generosity is that generosity puts the beneficiary under duties and expectations of gratitude, lowering their status vis à vis the benefactor.

Neither are animals our moral equals, nor is there an expectation that animals should be grateful for any benefits they receive from human beings.

However, even though expectations of gratitude play no role in our moral relations to animals, there can still be a duty on our part not to exalt ourselves over them, neither in the sense of taking an arrogant or contemptuous stance towards them, nor in the sense of going overboard in our beneficence out of delusions of grandeur. Granted, we can have no Kantian duty to recognise, and act in accordance with, the moral equality of beings who are not our moral equals. But why should there not instead be a duty to recognise, and act in accordance with, the fundamental moral *incomparability* of a being capable, and one incapable, of morality? The moral inequality between human beings and animals, as Cholbi has pointed out (2014, 348), lies not just in the fact that animals lack the potential for moral *goodness*, but also in that they lack the *propensity to evil.* Not standing under a moral law, they can be neither good nor bad when they go about their actions. Hence, they are neither morally better nor morally worse than human beings. But we fail to act in accordance with this fundamental moral inequality when we view animals as *morally worse* or *less deserving of their happiness* or *less important qua moral patients* than human beings. So we have a Kantian duty not to exalt ourselves above animals, at least not in any sense that would have us view ourselves as 'more worthy' of our happiness than they are of theirs (for, in contrast to human beings, they do not *need* to be worthy of their happiness). Kant's egalitarianism—the injunction not to exalt ourselves above others and hence not to be overbearingly beneficent upon them—can be drawn from the fundamental *inequality* between moral agents and non-agents, as much as from the fundamental *equality* between moral agents.

To be sure, the duty of non-exaltation will make different demands on us depending on whether we regard human beings or animals. To stay as close as possible to Kant, we can endorse his consideration that other human beings feel constrained or humiliated by overbearing beneficence (MM 6:448.21 25) and that we should strive not to embarrass others or otherwise lower their moral self-esteem. This is of no concern regarding animals who neither have nor need moral self-esteem in the first place. Still, the duty of non-exaltation asks us to be beneficent towards animals *only from the right stance.* We should act with a kind of humility which acknowledges that we are fallible, finite creatures, capable of doing good but always liable to doing wrong. We should not regard ourselves as would-be demigods of whose gracious assistance animals always need more and never less. The recognition of our own limitations puts a certain restriction on the *way* in which we should benefit animals, and this might impact the *extent* to which we try to benefit them as well. However, this restriction is less tight than that on our beneficence towards other human beings.

One might wonder why the move I suggest should apply only to our treatment of animals, and not to the whole rest of nature. Rocks and trees too are neither morally better nor morally worse than human beings, since they do not stand under the moral law. However, rocks and trees are not subjects of happiness, hence no moral patients according to Kantianism for Animals. In this moral framework, all specific duties towards others stem from the obligatory end of promoting their happiness (that is what makes them duties 'towards others'). More specific duties are essentially specifications as to *how* we should promote this obligatory end. Here, the moral inequality between human beings and animals gives rise to a specific qualification that we ought not to exalt ourselves above animals in our promotion of their happiness. But that does not imply that we have duties of respect to things that are incapable of happiness.

6.2 ADOPTING ANOTHER'S ENDS AS OUR OWN

Kant's system is built on the assumption that the 'others' to whom we have duties are rational beings in yet another way still. Consider that Kant asks us to 'adopt another's end as our own' (see MM 6:388.05–08; G 4:430.24–27; MM 6:340.03–05; Sect. 2.5). This formulation is not incidental. Kant purposely lays an emphasis on what others want for themselves, not on what we happen to think they should want. The reason for this emphasis is *not*, mind you, that instrumental practical reason has any kind of moral value which we must honour by furthering its ends and means. Kant makes it very clear that instrumental practical reason alone does not elevate the human being above other things in the world (CPrR 5:061.32–062.01). The reason why we ought to promote the ends of others is more banal: Our chief duty towards others is to promote their hedonic happiness, and the (non-moral) ends others set by means of instrumental practical reason serve as means to their hedonic happiness as well. So the most straightforward way to promote the happiness of others is usually to help along their own endeavours. But of course, this is only the case because others set their ends in an instrumental-rational way, as a means to their happiness. So despite the fact that instrumental practical reason has or produces no moral value in itself, it has a mediatory role to play in moral patienthood according to Kant's conception.

The idea has some intuitive pull that our chief duty towards animals, too, is to help along their own endeavours. It would be attractive if this feature of Kant's framework could be preserved in Kantianism for Animals. However, difficulties soon arise: Kant would deny that animals have any 'ends' whatsoever which we could adopt. So it is quite simply *impossible* to give them the Kantian treatment without amending Kant's picture to some extent. This becomes clear once we consider Kant's various remarks on animal behaviour (Sect. 6.3). However, I am going to argue that we can grant, within a Kantian framework, that animals have necessitating states that are non-conceptual, or 'conceptual' in another sense than Kant's, or which qualify as 'obscure', even if they are not proper 'ends' in Kant's technical sense (Sect. 6.4). So there is more than enough in terms of 'ends' we *could* adopt.

Furthermore, even if we grant that animals have such necessitating states, they do not stand in an instrumental-rational relation to their happiness. So even if we *could* help along their endeavours, the question remains why we *should*. In response, I am going to propose another line of reasoning in favour of concern for the necessitating states of animals. What matters most for Kant's ethics, I argue, is that another's ends serve an *indicative* function for their happiness. Though the motivations of animals may not serve this indicative function due to instrumental practical reason, they serve the same purpose based on biological functionality. In other words, animals may not *plan* to promote their own happiness by means of their actions, but many of their behaviours serve a biological function for their health and flourishing, which in turn stand in close relation to their happiness. The upshot of this argument is the view that the promotion of animal happiness is primarily a matter of helping along animals' own endeavours. This again gets us close to Kant's original picture. Before concluding, I want to take a moment to explore how much of Kant's specific list of ethical duties towards others we can transfer upon animals, based on the arguments in this chapter.

6.3   KANT'S DENIAL OF END-DIRECTED ANIMAL AGENCY

Although he never dedicated a separate piece of writing to the topic of animal behaviour, Kant has a somewhat detailed and coherent account of the differences between human and animal agency. The first and major difference, of course, is that human beings are transcendentally free, animals are not (A534/B562). Human beings can at least *consider* acting against their strongest natural impulse by acting from duty (CPrR 5:030.22–35). Acting from duty is however only possible through practical autonomy—the capacity to act on a self-imposed law independent of all natural laws. Animals, since they are not autonomous, lack this capacity. Their will is *necessitated* by sensibility, not merely *affected* by it (A534/B562). Along similar lines runs a claim recorded in the Mongrovius lecture notes: "Animals have no free choice, their actions being necessarily determined by their sensory impulses" (*Mongrovius* 29:611). Kant also calls this mode of agency the "animal power of choice (*arbitrium brutum*)" (A534/B562, see *Mongrovius* 29.611), as opposed to the human power of choice ("*arbitrium sensitivum*, yet not *brutum* but *liberum*", ibid.).

However, this view would still permit Kant to grant that animals have a limited form of instrumental practical reason. This would amount to the view that animals are ultimately bound to act on their sensory impulses, but are able to strategise to some extent, resisting momentary impulses for the sake of greater satisfaction later on. In fact, Kant acknowledges that there could conceivably be creatures who have all the capacities of instrumental practical reason, but who are still unfree (CPrR 5:449.04–07).

But in Kant's view, animals are not such creatures. This is clear in a passage from the *Collins* lecture notes: "Animals are necessitated *per stimulos*, so that a dog must eat if he is hungry and has something in front of him; but the human being, in the same situation, can restrain himself" (*Collins* 27:267). In Kant's own words from *Syllogismen*, a dog always acts according to "the natural connection which exists between its drives and its representations" (*Syllogismen* 2:060.08). That is to say, there is a hardwired behaviour for any sensation (which is all "representation" refers to at this point). And so, while human beings act on a complex system of ends and considerations, animals simply act on the next best impulse. Reason, even purely instrumental practical reason, does not enter the picture.

The absence of reason in animal behaviour has deeper implications: Not only can animals not strategise in their choice of means to preconceived ends, but they cannot pursue any *ends* at all. Acting for the sake of ends is itself an exercise of practical reason (MM 6:385.01–04). And this connection between reason and end-directed agency is not established by Kant arbitrarily. Reason is required for end-directed agency because acting on ends is essentially a *conceptual* capacity for Kant. Ends are always conceptually structured (see Guyer 2006, 349; Graband 2015, 16). This, in turn, is because ends are the *objects* of an intentional state, and they receive their object-shape from concepts. As much is clear from Kant's explicit definition: "An end is an *object* of free choice, the representation of which determines it to an action (by which the object is brought about)" (MM 6:384.33–34). The kind of object Kant has in mind here is a *logical* object of an intentional state, not necessarily a physical object in the natural world. To be sure, it *could* be a physical object, such as the cup of coffee I intend to produce by using the coffee maker. But the happiness of others, which we are supposed to make our end, is certainly not a physical object. What is important is rather that ends are clearly represented *some-things* picked out by means of concepts. They could be physical objects, substances, processes, states, properties, or really any referent of a clear representation.

However, Kant assumes that animals lack concepts (as McLear points out, McLear 2011, 4). Of course, this implies that animal actions cannot be guided by clear representations, even though awareness of perceptions may still influence their behaviour. Whatever animals do, they do it unknowingly, without a goal in view. As Kant puts it in the *Anthropology*, animals "manage provisionally" (Anth 7:196.26).

It appears, then, that Kant is committed to the following inference:

Argument against end-directed agency in animals

(1) Ends are objects.
(2) Representing objects requires concepts.
(3) Animals lack concepts.
(4) Therefore, animals cannot represent ends.

But if Kant accepts (4), how does he think animals do what they do? In a word, by *instinct*. Kant gives us a coherent picture of instinctive animal behaviour, even if it has attracted little attention in the literature.[2] It is a picture of animal behaviour that does entirely without end-directed agency or any other conceptual capacities. For the rest of this section, let me flesh out this picture before discussing alternative Kantian views in the next section.

---

[2] A rare exception is Katsafanas (2018).

In Kant's view, what sets the causes of animal actions apart from ends is their non-conceptual form. As he puts it in the third *Critique*: "The will, as the faculty of desire, is one of the many kinds of natural causes in the world, namely that which operates *in accordance with concepts*" (CPJ 5:172.04–06, emphasis added). So what is distinctive about the will is precisely that it operates with concepts. Kant then goes on to contrast the will with an example of a cause which operates *without* concepts and names animal instinct:

> everything that is represented as possible (or necessary) through a will is called practically possible (or necessary), in distinction from the physical possibility or necessity of an effect to which the cause is not determined to causality through concepts (but rather, as in the case of lifeless matter, through mechanism, *or, in the case of animals, through instinct*). (CPJ 5:172.06–11, emphasis added)

As this passage also reveals, Kant does not strictly equate instinct with mechanism. There is still something special about what Kant calls 'pathological necessitation' or 'psychological causality'. In psychological causality, not just physical bodies can be causal relata, but also representations (CPrR 5:069.30–31). The notion of 'representation' at work here is very broad: Mere sensations count too. Kant intends to reject what he takes to be Descartes's view, namely, that animals are mere bodily machines devoid of sensation (CPJ 5:464FN).[3] So even though animal action is caused by *non-conceptual* causes, they have *psychological* causes.

Kant's views about the causes of animal actions have certain implications concerning how those actions work. As we have already seen, end-directed human agency has some object clearly 'in view'. Agents can only be clearly aware of what they strive for if they represent it by relying on a concept. Without the concept of a cup of coffee, one cannot strive, with awareness, to obtain a cup of coffee. So instinct, as Kant also puts it, is "blind" (MM 6:376.22). Kant makes instinct's 'blindness' particularly salient in a passage from the *Anthropology*. Here he posits that instinct is

---

[3] Wild (2007) has pointed out that Descartes at times speaks of animals' "affects", which could suggest a form of sentience (Wild 2007, 165). How this is to be reconciled with Descartes's 'bêtes-machine' view is an open question. At any rate, Descartes's views on animals may have been more complicated than Kant acknowledges. Conversely, Kant's own view on animals as feeling cogs in the mechanism of nature may not go as far beyond Descartes's view as Kant supposes.

an in-between category between mere propensity and inclination. Propensity is the "subjective *possibility* of the emergence of a certain desire, which *precedes* the representation of its object" (Anth 7:265.21–22; see Rel 6:028FN). In other words, propensities are dispositions to desire that require no awareness of what we may come to desire. Kant's own example is the propensity to drink: We can be disposed to desire alcohol long before we try our first sip (Rel 6:028FN). Now, instinct is like a mere propensity in that it requires no clear representation of an object. The difference is merely that instinct already involves a *feeling* of desire: Instinct is "the inner necessitation of the faculty of desire to take possession of this object before one even knows it" (Anth 7:265.23–24, emphasis removed). One of Kant's examples is the instinct to procreate (Anth 7:265.25): An animal in heat *feels something* that causes it to act a certain way. But it does not have to think about any particular mate, or about mating, or about the young produced as a result. Desire is hardwired to activity.

To sum up, Kant does not believe that animals are things in nature like any other, but that they are subject to a specifically psychological form of causality. What distinguishes them from human beings, however, is their lack of concepts. Although animals may act on 'instincts', they cannot orient their behaviour on clear representations of objects in the way human beings do. This presents a challenge for those of us who want to include animals in Kant's account of moral concern, which is tied to the idea of 'adopting another's ends as our own'.

6.4   Animal 'Ends': Conceptual, Non-conceptual, 'Obscure'

It is not uncommon in Kantian animal ethics to accept a more generous picture of animal agency than Kant's. Korsgaard (2018), for instance, speaks of animals' 'ends' throughout her book. She even asserts that "an animal just is a being that takes its own functional good as the end of action" (Korsgaard 2018, 146). On another occasion, she asserts that in what she calls an 'instinctive' action, there always is the "animal's own purpose", such as "avoid the lion's attention" for an antelope who then chooses to duck in the grass (Korsgaard 2018, 42). A 'purpose', at this point, is not merely a biological function, in the way protecting the cornea is the biological function of an unintentional eye closure reflex. The animal's own purpose is something the animal itself represents as the goal of its action. The difference to the ends of a rational being is merely that rational beings are capable of choosing ends for themselves, while animals merely represent theirs.

How substantial a divergence from Kant does it represent if we assume that animals have 'ends'? It depends on what exactly we mean. As we have just seen in Sect. 6.3, Kant ties end-directed agency to conceptual capacities. When Kant speaks of 'ends', what he has in mind are object-shaped, conceptually structured representations that determine action. If we want to be able to claim that the Kantian injunction to adopt the ends of others applies to animals, it appears we have to disagree with Kant either on whether animals have concepts or on whether end-directed agency requires concepts. However, there is a third option. We can claim that animals have 'ends' in another sense than Kant's, but that these 'ends' can still play the role that matters for Kantian interpersonal ethics. In fact, we can make this move in several different ways. We can claim that animals have *non-conceptual necessitating states* or *necessitating states that are 'conceptual' in another sense than Kant's*, or so-called *obscure ends*. They do have a perspective on their own actions with which we can and should be morally concerned.

First, however, what would be the trouble with simply ascribing Kantian concepts to animals? The problem is that we would be attributing too much for it to be plausible. In order to have an end 'Kantian-style' to avoid a lion, antelopes would need to represent the lion by means of an 'empirical' concept, which is a concept whose content is an object given in experience. One important role of empirical concepts lies in allowing the subsumption of specific representations by the power of judgement (Heinz 2015). It allows a rational being to lend unity to what is initially a manifold of intuition. The other important role of empirical concepts is to be the building blocks of judgements, such as 'lions are dangerous'. But in order to play either role—for subsumption or for judgement—it is crucial that empirical concepts be *general*. That is, their application should be largely independent of context. Whoever can subsume a certain manifold of intuition under *lion* in one context should also be able to subsume the same manifold under *lion* in other contexts. And whoever has the concept of *lion* must be able to form and understand various judgements about lions—not just 'lions are dangerous', but also 'lions are to be avoided', or 'lions avoid fire', provided the concepts are known. In the language of analytic philosophy, having Kantian concepts is a capacity with a very strong Generality Constraint (McLear 2016, 182; see Evans 1982). That is to say, to have a Kantian concept is to be able to combine it with other concepts, or with other manifolds of intuition, with only few limitations.[4]

Ascribing a capacity with such a strong Generality Constraint to animals like antelopes is implausible. If antelopes do have a concept of *lion*, a concept of *danger*, and presumably some other concepts too, it seems that they only use their conceptual vocabulary in tightly restricted ways. They seem to keep judging that lions are dangerous, but they do not combine this judgement with other judgements in a way that would enable them to develop more elaborate strategies of avoiding lions than merely by ducking in the grass. If antelopes could flexibly recombine concepts, we should expect much more productivity and systematicity from their thought (see Beck 2012, 222ff.). The more plausible view, by far, is that antelope thoughts and actions are not structured in a way *Kant* would accept as conceptual. They may be capable of 'conceptual' thought in another sense of the term, but it is uncontroversial that they lack concepts *in Kant's sense*. And since Kantian 'ends' are structured by Kantian concepts, it is implausible to ascribe Kantian 'ends' to animals.

But of course, Kantian 'ends' are merely a species of a larger class of action-determining or necessitating states. So even if we deny that animals pursue 'ends' in Kant's technical sense, we can ascribe to animals 'ends' in the sense of some other, non-conceptual species of necessitating state. Of course, the *instincts* Kant ascribes to animals already fit this description, since they are non-conceptual necessitating states. However, the vocabulary of instinct can obscure the true complexity of animal behaviour. Within the broad class of 'instincts', we might find necessitating states which consist of discrete parts that can be systematically recombined to a certain extent, or they might be based on some capacity to stably discriminate between Xs and non-Xs (Beck 2012, 222). Certain animals may even be capable of drawing inferences and thinking in a means-ends-rational way within certain contexts (so-called islands of rationality, Hurley 2003, 2006). In short, animals' necessitating states may have a lot more to them than Kant's account of instinct would have it, all without Kantian concepts.

Another way to expand Kant's view of animal agency is to grant that animals are capable of a non-conceptual mode of objective perceptual

---

[4] One may grant that even competent users of Kantian concepts may be unable to grasp nonsensical or contradictory judgements using the concepts. So the Generality Constraint on Kantian concepts is not infinitely strong. Still, within the bounds of meaningfulness and consistency, a competent user should be able to use Kantian concepts flexibly.

awareness (see McLear 2011, 2016, 2020). For philosophers interested in Kant's views on perception, to claim that object perception is possible without concepts may seem problematic. After all, Kant gives great weight to the claim that concepts, and ultimately the categories, are a condition of the possibility of object perception (Kitcher 1984; Naragon 1990). However, we need to be clear about what *kind* of perceptual object awareness we are concerned with. As McLear points out, Kant himself at times asserts that animals are in some ways *acquainted* with objects (McLear 2011, 5). This acquaintance comes in the form of what Kant calls 'obscure' or 'unconscious' representations (*Jäsche* 9:33.25–26; see McLear 2011, 6). Such representations provide some sensory awareness, but do not enable us to individuate the object. For example, we might be aware of a violin's sound in an orchestra, but still be unable to pick it out individually (McLear 2011, 6). Similarly, an antelope may be aware of a lion in its environment without however being able to *individuate* the lion in a way that would allow, say, reidentification of the lion in another environment. But if animals can have such 'obscure' representations, we may as well grant them 'obscure ends' structured by just these representations. For instance, an antelope may want to get away from lion-environments, though not from individuated lions. So even within the restrictions of a Kantian philosophy of perception, we can accommodate a more sophisticated view of animal behaviour than Kant himself advances.

To sum up, I have suggested that animals do not plausibly pursue 'ends' in Kant's narrow, technical sense, but they can still have necessitating states that are non-conceptual, or 'conceptual' in another sense than Kant's, or 'obscure'. There is enough here in the way of 'ends' that we *could* adopt if a Kantian framework demanded it.

A second issue remains, however: Even if animals have 'ends' of some kind, why should these 'ends' concern us? If animals' ends are to be morally relevant in the same way as the ends of Kantian rational beings, they need to be relevantly similar. Here, the crucial question is what makes our ends 'valuable' in the sense that others have a duty to adopt them. Korsgaard, with her influential interpretation of Kantian ethics, begins this explanation from the perspective of the moral patient. As we saw in Sect. 4.3, Korsgaard argues that we confer goodness upon our ends by rationally choosing and pursuing them. Her argument then revolves around showing that we must grant a version of this goodness-conferring capacity ('end-in-itselfhood' in Korsgaard's sense) to all animals, since animals pursue their natural ends in much the same way as we do (Korsgaard 2004, 102–6, 2018, 143f.).

By contrast, the reading of Kant's ethics I have suggested focuses steadfastly on the moral agent: We have a duty to adopt the ends of others, not because of any morally important feature of those ends themselves, but because our duty is to promote another's happiness. The *ends* of human beings should concern us only because we can presume that these ends point towards the subject's *happiness* in an instrumentally rational way. We set most of our ends merely as means to further ends, and the ultimate (non-moral) end is our own happiness. Thus, if we are looking for means to promote the happiness of others, we are well advised to use their ends as indicators.

Kant emphasises that we can be beneficent to others "only according to the concepts of him whom I would like to render a benefit" (MM 6:454.20–21). Fittingly, however, he at the very same time puts a restriction on his own demand that we let others judge for themselves what makes them happy:

> I cannot be beneficent to anyone according to my concepts of happiness (*except for children during their minority or the mentally disturbed*), but only according to the concepts of him whom I would like to render a benefit by urging a gift upon him. (MM 6:454.18–21, emphasis removed and added)

Kant's point, evidently, is that only certain adult human beings are fully competent judges of their own happiness. Only with regard to these specific human beings should we understand our duty of beneficence to demand that we help along the realisation of their own ends. Of course, we can and should disagree with Kant about the true capacities of those of us who are young or have disabilities, and about the extent to which they should get to determine the course of their own lives. For animals, however, the case seems fairly clear: It is implausible that animals set their ends (in whatever sense of the term) in an instrumentally rational way across the board, so that they all serve the ultimate end of happiness. At best, certain animals are capable of instrumental reasoning within certain contexts (see again Hurley 2003, 2006).

According to this understanding of Kant's ethics, however, it is not truly instrumental rationality that does the most work. The instrumentally rational relation that connects our ends to our happiness itself matters only because it makes our ends *indicators* of our happiness. The question is hence not whether animals' ends stand in an instrumentally rational relation to their happiness, but whether they *indicate* what makes animals happy. And they clearly do, at least to a significant extent. There is actually a way of making this point in a distinctively Kantian way. It consists of two steps: first, in distinguishing between two types of functionality, practical and natural. Though animal behaviours may not 'aim' at happiness in the practical sense (so that happiness is the highest end in an instrumentally rational hierarchy of ends), they can still 'aim' at happiness, or at least at some of its prerequisites, as a matter of natural or biological functionality. Secondly, the solution consists in acknowledging that animal behaviours *actually do* serve biological purposes closely related to the animal's hedonic happiness. As I will argue in the remainder of this section, both steps are readily possible within Kant's framework. The upshot is that we should think of beneficence towards animals largely as the promotion of their own 'ends', not because animals choose these ends as means to their happiness, but because they serve the same indicative function for biological reasons.[5]

Kant himself devotes much attention to the question whether there is purposiveness in nature in the second part of the *Critique of the Power of Judgment*, called the *Critique of the Teleological Power of Judgment*. He discusses 'relative purposiveness', which we might nowadays call ecological functionality, as well as 'internal purposiveness', which translates more closely to biological functionality (CPrR 5:366f.). Kant subsumes both types of functionality under the general label 'end of nature' (*Naturzweck*). Though Kant rejects realism about natural ends (CPJ 5:394.13), he vindicates a teleological perspective on nature on the grounds that "because of the peculiar constitution of my cognitive faculties I cannot judge about the possibility of those things and their generation except by thinking of a cause for these that acts in accordance with intentions" (CPrR 5:397.34–398.02). Hence, though Kant does not believe that ecological functionality is a matter of anyone's intentions, let alone God's, he considers teleological judgement to be indispensable for human beings.

---

[5] Another upshot here is that even if a machine should 'want' anything, this does not automatically give us a duty of beneficence towards it on the Kantian-for-Animals view. It is not the *wanting* that gives us a duty to promote the ends of others, but the obligatory end of the happiness of others. Hence, only if machines were capable of happiness—on a hedonic conception of happiness—and only if their wants pointed to their happiness, would Kantianism for Animals demand that we promote the ends of machines.

To be sure, the perspective on animals we need in order to include them in Kantian moral concern has little to do with their status as a 'relative means' for other things in nature. What counts instead are the functional relations between animals' ends on the one hand, and their happiness on the other. Even if there may not be an instrumental-rational hierarchy of practical ends that leads from momentary actions all the way to the ultimate end of happiness, there can be a string of biological functions of the same extent. In this sense, animals do 'pursue' their happiness, even if they cannot *represent* their own happiness in general as a practical end.

In more contemporary language, we can say that many animal behaviours and the necessitating states that cause them serve a *biological* function for prerequisites of the animal's happiness. For example, food approach and wanting-food are biologically functional for nutrition, and nutrition of course contributes to hunger satisfaction and health, both of which typically promote the happiness of the animal. So even though a certain *practical-functional* order is absent in what many animals want, there is more than enough of a *biological-functional* order to make animals' necessitating states important moral guideposts for us.

When it comes to the claim that animal behaviours actually do serve biological functions closely related to their happiness, Kant would not have to disagree. In fact, in the *Religion* he claims that human beings have an entirely pre-rational mode of self-love, which he terms 'physical and merely mechanical self-love' (Rel 6:026.13, see Rinne 2018, 22). This mode of self-love promotes unwitting behaviours that are biologically conducive to self-preservation, species propagation, and community with other human beings (Rel 6:026.14–18). Nothing stops Kant from endorsing the same view with regard to animals.

What is more, to some extent Kant already associates instinct with happiness, as a well-known passage from the *Groundwork* reveals:

> Now in a being that has reason and a will, if the proper end of nature were its preservation, its welfare, in a word its happiness, then nature would have hit upon a very bad arrangement in selecting the reason of the creature to carry out its purpose. For all the actions that the creature has to perform for this purpose, and the whole rule of its conduct, would be marked out for it far more accurately by instinct. (G 4:395.04–16)

To be precise, Kant here only claims that nature could have created *some* happiness-conducive instinct in human beings, not that the *actual* instincts of animals produce their happiness. His main point is that if the purpose of reason lied in the natural world, that purpose would have been better served by some hardwired natural mechanism. Still, Kant's view would easily allow him to claim that animal actions typically *do* serve to produce their happiness, or at least prerequisites of their happiness such as self-preservation and species-typical community.

To add a caveat, note that the argument in this section does not demand that we promote *just any* animal impulse, just as Kant himself does not demand that we help along the *next best* end others happen to have. In certain cases, the actions of animals and human beings might fail to indicate what makes them happy overall. For instance, an obese animal may pursue food intake too vigorously. This is a perfectly functional type of behaviour, but in this instance, it is a threat to health. A threat to health is usually a threat to happiness. So we ought not to help along this behaviour. Within these reasonable restrictions, however, we should take an animal's own ends as guideposts for our beneficence.

Before moving on, let me address a potential worry. The move of the present section is to liken the *biological* functionality of certain animal behaviours to the *practical* functionality of human actions as Kant thinks of them. This might be a red flag to some Kantians, and addressing it may well be useful for animal ethicists too. As Altman warns:

> If natural purposiveness is what is morally relevant, then all living organisms are directly morally considerable because things may frustrate or promote their teleological development. Although most environmental ethicists accept this, it takes us a long way from Kant. (Altman 2011, 25f.)

The reason it takes us a long way from Kant is that for Kant, moral concern hinges on the mutual sharing of the moral law. Altman is right to caution against acting as though an internal biological-functional structure could simply replace the moral law in Kant's picture of interpersonal moral obligation. So I should emphasise that this is *not* the move I am advocating. What I have proposed (in Chap. 5) is that we can replace Kant's second-personal view of interpersonal moral obligation with a thoroughly first-personal one. According to this view, what gives rise to our ethical duties towards others is our own autonomy, paired with the fact that others are subjects of hedonic happiness. To this line of reasoning, the present section adds an argument why a good Kantian agent should pay attention to animal *behaviours* and *necessitating states*. Though these may not be part of an elaborate, instrumental-rational project conceived to promote the subject's happiness (as Kant thinks human actions are), they still serve biological purposes that relate to the animal's happiness. So this chapter's arguments do not imply that the line of moral concern is to be drawn at biological-functional structures. Nor does it assume that any kind of inherent value or value-conferring power attaches to biological functionality. Rather, they imply that in our treatment of beings with a happiness at stake, the biological functionality of their behaviours gives us reason to adopt their 'ends' as our own, at least within certain reasonable restrictions.

With these considerations ends the core argument for Kantianism for Animals. I have argued that the formulations of the Categorical Imperative do not present a serious obstacle to the inclusion of animals, since they do not settle the issue of who deserves moral concern. We need not tamper with this central part of Kant's ethical system. What we must indeed change is Kant's understanding of the directionality of ethical duties. I have argued that we can think of duties 'towards' others simply as duties that derive from the obligatory end of the happiness of others. This end is obligatory because it is a part of the highest good in the world, one that we can actually bring about by means of our actions. But animals' happiness belongs to the highest good in the world, since it is a happiness that is not tainted by vice. Therefore, on this amended Kantian view, we have duties towards animals. The final step was then to remove the last anthropocentrisms from Kant's system, particularly concerning the notion of duties of respect and regard for the self-chosen ends of the individual. These features do not need to be purged from Kant's system, however, but can be accommodated in an animal-friendly way.

Along the way, I hope to have conveyed a glimpse into the kind of ethical outlook that Kantianism for Animals can bring to the table in animal ethics. It provides an account of what it means for ethical duties to be directed 'towards' an animal, and of what we ought to do, expressed at different levels of generality (adopting specific ends of others, adopting practical-emotional stances, promoting happiness). Having developed the Kantianism for Animals framework in general, let me try to situate it in the theoretical landscape of animal ethics and highlight what makes the framework distinctive. That is the purpose of the next chapter.

References

Altman, Matthew C. 2011. *Kant and applied ethics: The uses and limits of Kant's practical philosophy*. Malden, MA: Wiley-Blackwell.

Baron, Marcia W. 2002. Love and respect in the Doctrine of Virtue. In *Kant's Metaphysics of Morals: Interpretative essays*, ed. Mark Timmons, 391–407. Oxford: Oxford University Press.

Beck, Jacob. 2012. Do animals engage in conceptual thought? *Philosophy Compass* 7: 218–229.

Cholbi, Michael. 2014. A direct Kantian duty to animals. *The Southern Journal of Philosophy* 52: 338–358.

Evans, Gareth. 1982. *The varieties of reference*. Oxford: Clarendon Press.

Fahmy, Melissa S. 2007. Understanding Kant's Duty of Respect as a Duty of Virtue. *Journal of Moral Philosophy* 10(6): 723–740.

Graband, Claudia. 2015. *Klugheit bei Kant*. Berlin: De Gruyter.

Guyer, Paul, ed. 2006. *The Cambridge companion to Kant and modern philosophy*. Cambridge: Cambridge University Press.

Heinz, Marion. 2015. Begriff, empirischer. In *Kant-Lexikon*, ed. Marcus Willaschek, Jürgen Stolzenberg, Georg Mohr, and Stefano Bacin, 240–241. Berlin: De Gruyter.

Hurley, Susan. 2003. Animal action in the space of reasons. *Mind & Language* 18: 231–257.

Hurley, Susan. 2006. Making sense of animals. In *Rational animals?*, ed. Susan Hurley and Matthew Nudds, 136–172. Oxford: Oxford University Press.

Katsafanas, Paul. 2018. The emergence of the drive concept and the collapse of the animal/human divide. In *Oxford philosophical concepts: Animals*, ed. Peter Adamson and G. Fay Edwards, 239–267. Oxford: Oxford University Press.

Kitcher, Patricia. 1984. Kant's real self. In *Self and nature in Kant's philosophy*, ed. Allen W. Wood. Ithaca, NY: Cornell University Press.

Korsgaard, Christine M. 2004. Fellow creatures. The Tanner Lectures on Human Values.

Korsgaard, Christine M. 2018. *Fellow creatures: Our obligations to the other animals*. Oxford: Oxford University Press.

McLear, Colin. 2011. Kant on animal consciousness. *Philosophers' Imprint* 11: 1–16.

McLear, Colin. 2016. Getting acquainted with Kant. In *Kantian nonconceptualism*, 171–197. London: Palgrave Macmillan.

McLear, Colin. 2020. Animals and objectivity. In *Kant and animals*, ed. John J. Callanan and Lucy Allais, 42–64. Oxford: Oxford University Press.

Naragon, Steve. 1990. Kant on Descartes and the brutes. *Kant-Studien* 81: 1–23.

Rinne, Pärttyli. 2018. *Kant on love*. Berlin: De Gruyter.

Vogt, Katja M. 2009. Duties to others: Demands and limits. In *Kant's ethics of virtue*, ed. Monika Betzler, 219–244. Berlin: De Gruyter.

Wild, Markus. 2007. Die anthropologische Differenz: Der Geist der Tiere in der frühen Neuzeit bei Montaigne, Descartes und Hume. Berlin: De Gruyter.

Open Access   This chapter is licensed under the terms of the Creative Commons Attribution 4.0 International License (http://creativecommons.org/licenses/by/4.0/), which permits use, sharing, adaptation, distribution and reproduction in any medium or format, as long as you give appropriate credit to the original author(s) and the source, provide a link to the Creative Commons licence and indicate if changes were made.

The images or other third party material in this chapter are included in the chapter's Creative Commons licence, unless indicated otherwise in a credit line to the material. If material is not included in the chapter's Creative Commons licence and your intended use is not permitted by statutory regulation or exceeds the permitted use, you will need to obtain permission directly from the copyright holder.

CHAPTER 7

Kantianism for Animals: The Framework in Five Claims

7.1 Duties from Autonomy

If we take the steps advocated in the last three chapters, Kantianism for Animals results. It is a Kantian ethical framework that includes animals in moral concern in the same way and on the same grounds as human beings. I want to suggest that it is also the closest thing to Kant's ethics that progressive animal ethicists can accept in good conscience. The point of this framework, however, is not just to be a cruelty-free substitute to the 'real thing' (although there is nothing wrong with a good substitute). The point is that an approach that makes certain Kantian commitments might be positively helpful and interesting for animal ethicists. At this point, it will help to pause for a moment and consider an overview of Kantianism for Animals, particularly concerning the points that distinguish it from dominant approaches to animal ethics.

For convenience's sake, let me divide this overview into five claims: Kantianism for Animals is a moral framework which grounds duties in autonomy, considers duties to be primary over moral rights, recognises duties to self and duties to others, asks us to reconcile practical love for others with a maxim of non-exaltation, and which ties the moral worth of actions to their incentives. In the following chapters, I will then go further into detail and discuss some potential uses of Kantianism for Animals regarding more specific ethical questions.

© The Author(s) 2022
N. D. Müller, *Kantianism for Animals*, The Palgrave Macmillan
Animal Ethics Series,
https://doi.org/10.1007/978-3-031-01930-2_7

To see what is distinctive about the Kantian-for-Animals framework, we should first of all consider how it grounds duties in autonomy. Recall my argument from Chap. 4: Kant's account of moral concern—of how we ought to treat others—does not follow directly from the Formula of Humanity or any other formulation of the Categorical Imperative. Attempts to ground moral concern in the special value Kant accords to rational beings lead into fallacy. This special value can only explain why we are due moral *esteem*—an approving acknowledgement of our potential to be morally good—but not why we are due moral *concern*, such as in the form of beneficence. The proper place of moral concern in Kant's system is in the doctrine of obligatory ends, which is grounded in the doctrine of the highest good in the world. With only a slight amendment to these two connected doctrines, we can progress to the materially specific duties we have towards ourselves and others, including duties towards animals.

This argument has an immediate upshot: Whatever we must do to Kant's system in order to make it include animals as moral patients, the parts of it which he establishes in the *Groundwork* stay broadly intact. This is just not where the issue lies. I have argued in Chaps. 4 and 5 that we must differ from Kant when it comes to the conditions of 'duties towards' and the conception of animals themselves. We must deflate Kant's partially second-personal approach to duties towards others to a purely first-personal one, and we must grant more complex capacities to animals than Kant himself would have allowed. But none of this is particularly destructive to Kant's system.

Entire branches of Kant's moral philosophy remain unchanged in Kantianism for Animals. This is true, most importantly, for Kant's views on the relation between moral duties, autonomy, and free will. Kant asserts that the rational being must think of herself as free in order to act (G 4:448.09–11), and being free entails the capacity to act on a self-imposed law rather than merely according to the laws of nature (CPrR 5:093.32–094.02). This autonomously imposed law is the moral law from which our ethical duties spring (G 1.110.11–15), and heteronomy is the origin of all false principles of morality (G 4:441.01–02). Kantianism for Animals affirms all of these claims.

Therefore, Kantianism for Animals allots a crucial role to our own autonomy—understood as the capacity to act on a self-imposed law, which is the moral law. We could put the view in the following words:

Duties from autonomy

Ethical duties derive their bindingness from the autonomously imposed moral law.

Autonomy plays the role of the *normative basis* of our duties—it accounts for their bindingness. Autonomy is *ipso facto* the capacity that accounts for our having duties. Contrast this with a claim Kantianism for Animals does not advance: that autonomy is a trait that, in virtue of its own value, makes its bearers particularly precious or to-be-protected, directly giving rise to moral claims. Kantianism for Animals does not rest on such a valorisation of autonomy. Moral claims do not arise directly from any supposed value of autonomy, but are merely the correlatives of the duties of others, which in turn arise from autonomy.

In fact, Kantianism for Animals stands out for how little it emphasises the notion of the *value of individuals* in general when it derives its duties. What it means for animals to 'matter', to 'deserve moral concern', is *not* for them to exhibit some substantive moral value to which moral agents must be receptive. Rather, to 'matter' is to figure in the content of rational beings' duties in a certain way, namely as a being with a happiness at stake. And so, the previous chapters have not contained arguments to the effect that animals, or their pleasures and pains, or their lives, exhibit any substantive moral 'value' (or value-conferring capacity) from which we must then derive our duties. Rather, I have been concerned with the content of the duties of moral agents and whether animals can figure in this content in a particular way.

Kantianism for Animals differs from orthodox Kantian theory in that it does not view the moral law as essentially *co-legislated* by all rational beings. There is no 'second-personal' moral authority according to this theory at all. At best, statements to the effect that the moral law is 'co-legislated' by all rational beings are a shorthand to convey that it is not *individual human beings* who make moral rules, but that the moral law is a law of pure practical reason, a capacity regarding which all finite rational beings are equal. So all rational beings legislate *alike*, but not *together*. Taken literally, we do not co-legislate or even just share the moral law—we stand under moral laws with the same content each, which we have each autonomously self-imposed. Others—be they human beings or animals—can help to determine the content of our duties, but they cannot make these duties binding or lift them off our shoulders.

Its emphasis on autonomy sets Kantianism for Animals apart from virtually all prominent approaches to animal ethics. Of course, there is a contrast to any form of utilitarianism that is based on an axiology of utility (such as value hedonism). Its emphasis on autonomy as the normative basis of our duties also sets it starkly apart from sentimentalist, virtue-ethical, care-ethical, and contractualist approaches.

Perhaps more surprisingly, however, even self-avowedly 'deontological' and Kantian approaches to animal ethics have given notions of value great explanatory importance in the derivation of duties.[1] Regan relies so heavily on the notion of 'inherent value' that it has been called his "heaviest theoretical weapon" (Narveson 1987a, 197, 1987b, 37). Indeed, the notion of inherent value is crucial to Regan's argument at several points. For instance, he uses it to demarcate the realm of rights-bearers (Regan 2004, 243ff.), as well as to clarify his notion of 'respect' (Regan 2004, 248). And even Wood and Korsgaard, both card-carrying Kantians, rely on readings of Kant's arguments in the *Groundwork* according to which these arguments revolve around the value (or value-conferring capacity) of 'ends in themselves'. As discussed in Sect. 4.3, Wood and Korsgaard differ when it comes to the source of this value. For Wood, it is a preexisting, substantive value which rational beings can only *detect*. For Korsgaard, it is a value *created* by rational beings through acts of choice. For both, however, moral patienthood is a matter of exhibiting some value, and moral concern is a matter of reacting to that value in the right way. So even among 'deontological' and expressly Kantian views in animal ethics, Kantianism for Animals stands out for the way it derives its duties—as if by the motto 'duty first, not value first'.

7.2   The Primacy of Duties over Rights and Claims

Kantianism for Animals treats *duties* as the primary unit of moral prescription. As we have just seen, duties are binding not because they respond to some inherent value of individuals, but because they derive from an autonomously imposed moral law. From this emphasis on autonomy also arises the primacy of duties over moral rights. Moral rights exist only in virtue of their correlative duties (explanatory primacy), we can only know about our moral rights by deriving them from our duties (epistemic primacy), and moral rights derive all their bindingness from their correlative duties (normative primacy). Not vice versa. The same holds for 'claims', even if they are conceived of as a weaker kind of demand than rights. To sum up:

---

[1] Regan never called himself a Kantian, but he did claim to belong to a "Kantian tradition" (Regan 2004, xvii; see also Regan 2003, 77).

Duties over rights and claims

Duties have explanatory, epistemic, and normative primacy over moral rights and claims.

Although animal ethicists often associate Kant with rights theory, it is actually not uncommon for Kantians to be sceptical of the very notion of a moral right due to the primacy of duties over rights (see e.g. Mohr 2010). If moral rights are merely a roundabout way of speaking about duties, we might as well speak about duties directly to ward off confusions and distractions.

The primacy of duties over rights sets Kantianism for Animals in apparent contrast to Regan, who calls his own view the 'rights view'. However, it is not as though Regan ever explicitly committed to the explanatory, epistemic, and normative primacy of rights over duties. This would require adopting a substantive account of moral bindingness or goodness, which is exactly what Regan's method of ethical argument is designed to avoid. He begins not from a substantive account of the right and the good, but from a series of candidate moral theories that are simply posited and then tested for consistency, adequacy of scope, precision, and conformity with intuitions (Regan 2004, 131–136). Although to my knowledge, Regan never made this explicit, his method is perfectly compatible with a Moorean scepticism vis à vis substantive accounts of goodness. And here lies the true underlying difference between Kantianism for Animals and Regan: Regan's view does not commit to a substantive view about the nature of duties and rights (only to a certain method and place to draw the line of moral consideration), Kantianism for Animals does. The contrast here is not between believers of different faiths, but between a believer and an agnostic. Despite all differences in vocabulary and emphasis, then, to some extent we can think of Kantianism for Animals as a complement to Regan more than as a competitor. It provides a substantive account of the nature of duties, which Regan avoids.

The reason why Kantianism for Animals considers duties to be primary is that it is connected to Kant's account of moral bindingness as arising from autonomy. Duties only bind us because they are derived from the autonomously imposed moral law. If moral rights were to be more than mere correlates of our duties, there would have to be some authority by whose power we are bound to respect them. But such an authority would lie outside of the moral agent herself and would thus be heteronomous. For this reason, moral rights cannot be primary in Kantianism for Animals, and indeed it is doubtful whether talk of 'moral rights' is useful in this framework at all. We may as well cut out the middleman and talk about ethical duties.

The preoccupation with notions of duty does not restrict the level of generality at which Kantianism for Animals can issue its prescriptions. This level of generality corresponds to the description of the case. If we consider ourselves merely as human beings who share the world with others who pursue their own happiness, our duty is simply to 'promote the happiness of others and our own moral perfection'. But the more facts about ourselves and others we take into consideration, the more specific our duties become. However, Kant's own aspiration is not to answer moral questions with quasi-scientific precision (Wood 2007, 54–57). In the particular situation, we always need our own capacity for moral judgement. Moral philosophy can only direct us towards the right kinds of considerations. Often, the way in which it does this is by highlighting the emotional-practical *stance* we ought to take towards ourselves and others—avoid arrogance, be beneficent, do not be cruel, and so on. Or it can help us select general maxims in accordance with duty. For this reason, Kantianism for Animals does not fit the stereotype of an absolutist 'deontological' approach that obtusely insists on the observation of generally conceived rules irrespective of the particular situation (which is a description Kant's moral philosophy in general does not fit (Timmermann 2015, 85–88)).

Another upshot of the primacy of duties is that there can be duties which do *not* correspond to any rights. As we saw in Sect. 2.6, Kant refers to these duties as 'meritorious'. This is one of the ways in which Kantianism for Animals goes beyond traditional animal rights philosophy and offers resources to make up for some of its gaps. As philosophers of various backgrounds have argued, the notion of an 'animal right' is too narrow to capture the richness and complexity of our moral relations with animals. To name some influential examples, Diamond has called for the notion of a 'fellow creature', in analogy to our 'fellow human beings' (Diamond 1978). Gruen calls on animal ethicists to pay more attention to moral *capabilities* such as empathy, rather than moral principles (Gruen 2015). Benton calls for *solidarity* with animals, in addition to the mere 'safety net' of rights (Benton 1996). These calls are motivated, in one way or another, by the insight that from moral rights alone, we can only construct a quasi-legalistic hydraulics of competing claims, and this often does not make for an adequate or helpful representation of the moral landscape. Kantianism for Animals takes an interesting place in this discussion. By prioritising duties over rights, incorporating duties that do not correspond to rights, and tying duties to various emotions, it opens the view to a fuller picture of the moral landscape than is associated with traditional animal rights philosophy. To some extent, we can turn this into a defence of animal rights philosophy: It is not necessarily connected to an impoverished representation of the moral landscape, provided we understand rights as mere correlates of duties and then focus on the richer vocabulary of duties. However, the vocabulary provided by Kantianism for Animals might itself be helpful to further articulate ideas of fellow-being, entangled empathy, and solidarity.

7.3   Duties to Self and Others

Kantianism for Animals is unique in contemporary animal ethics in that it recognises two types of duties, namely to self and others:

Duties to self and others

We have a duty to others to promote their happiness, and a duty to self to promote our own moral perfection.

As we have seen in Chap. 5, Kantianism for Animals takes the directionality of our duties to be a matter of duty-content. Duties that derive from the obligatory end of the happiness of others are called duties 'towards' others, while those that derive from our own moral perfection are duties 'towards' self. There is no requirement of mutual 'constraint' because the bindingness of moral duties rests only on the autonomy of the moral agent.

Our duties towards others demand that we promote their happiness. The account of happiness presupposed is broadly hedonistic—to be happy is to experience maximum pleasantness. This implies that moral patients on the Kantian-for-Animals view must be capable of feeling pleasure. Hence, this framework draws the line of moral concern in a familiar place, namely at sentience.[2] However, the agency of others plays a crucial role for the way in which we ought to *promote* their happiness: We ought to use another's own actions and behaviours as guideposts for our attempts at

---

[2] If Godfrey-Smith is right that sentience comes in degrees (Godfrey-Smith 2021), this of course complicates the picture. As it stands, Kantianism for Animals has no clearer response to this gradation than other approaches to animal ethics. This is an area where the framework stands in need of further development.

beneficence. In Kant's words, "what they may count as belonging to their happiness is left to their own judgement" (MM 6:388.08–09).

Of course, the demand that we promote the happiness of others, including animals, does not make Kantianism for Animals particularly unique in the landscape of animal ethics (though it is distinctive among Kantian approaches in demanding beneficence for animals *on the same grounds* as beneficence towards humans). What does make Kantianism for Animals unique, however, is that it also recognises duties towards self. They stem from the obligatory end of our own moral perfection—which is another feature which generally sets Kantianism apart from utilitarianism (Timmermann 2005a, 252). What does concern for our own 'moral perfection' amount to? Kant distinguishes between two types of duties that follow from this obligatory end: duties that pertain to us as animal beings and duties that pertain to us purely as moral beings. Among the former, Kant lists the duty not to commit prudential suicide (MM 6:422.03), not to overindulge in sexual urges (MM 6:242.10), nor in drugs and food (MM 6:427.02–03). Kant's overall point is that we ought to keep ourselves, as natural beings, in a shape that is serviceable to our moral capacities. This requires, of course, that we are alive. It also requires that we retain the ability to overcome our urges if necessary.

Among the latter type of duty, Kant lists duties against lying (MM 6:429.02), against being overly frugal (MM 6:432.02), and against servility (MM 6:434.20). Here, the central idea is that we ought to act in accordance with the *esteem* we are due as moral beings (see Chap. 4). At this point, Kant presupposes that we already accept, on independent grounds, that lying is wrong. The additional problem he points out is that by lying, we sacrifice a clear conscience for the sake of our happiness and make ourselves an object of contempt in our own eyes: "For the dishonour (to be an object of moral contempt) that accompanies it also accompanies a liar, like his shadow" (MM 6:429.11–13). So quite distinctly from other prohibitions of lying, there also exists a duty not to lie because we should avoid having to hold ourselves in contempt. The other two duties are more straightforward: By being overly frugal, we fail to acknowledge that we can only act on our moral capacities if certain basic needs are met. By being servile towards others, we fail to see that we are their moral equals.

The other side of the coin is that we *only* have duties of moral self-perfection towards ourselves. We do not have a duty of self-love, or to secure even just a fair share of goods for ourselves. To promote our own happiness may be our inclination, but it is only other people's duty. Hence,

Kantianism for Animals has a strong tendency towards altruism, or even sacrifice. This tendency is restricted only by the indirect duty to secure the minimum of happiness we need in order to remain moral agents at all, which is a duty of moral self-perfection (see G 4:399.03–07; MM 6:388.26–28).

That there are duties towards both self and others has another mentionable upshot: Kantianism for Animals can retain the notion of an 'amphiboly of moral concepts of reflection' (see Chap. 3). That is, we can confuse a duty of one type for a duty of the other type. For example, our duty to cultivate our capacity for sympathy is still a duty towards self, since it is about our own moral perfection. But it may *appear* to us like a duty towards others. That is a confusion. The crucial difference to Kant is that the 'amphiboly' does not need to *explain away* what appears to us like a duty towards animals. Since there indeed do exist duties towards animals, we may as well trust our ordinary feelings of obligation towards them. But if all we are concerned with is a duty to cultivate our own sympathy, and we take *this* to be a duty towards someone else, animal or human, we have fallen prey to a confusion.

7.4   PRACTICAL LOVE AND NON-EXALTATION

Kantianism for Animals preserves many of the main distinctions of Kant's taxonomy of duties in the *Doctrine of Virtue*. We have already seen the distinction between duties to self and others at work. Another major distinction, between perfect and imperfect duties, is preserved too. This distinction does not pick up on whether duties allow for arbitrary exceptions on the grounds of inclination—no duty does that. The difference is rather that perfect duties are so specific that whenever we *can* observe them, we *must*. Imperfect duties are broader and apply to many situations, so that we must choose *when* and *how* to observe them, but observe them we must. To make this choice, we must consider our imperfect duties in context with all other duties. For example, our duty not to be arrogant is a perfect duty. Whenever we are tempted to be arrogant towards others, we must resist. Our duty of beneficence, by contrast, is imperfect. There are many situations and many ways in which to help others, and we must choose carefully when and how to do it. So our task is to figure out, in reflecting on our various duties, how to best help others while also observing our other duties. Another general distinction Kantianism for Animals adopts from Kant is that between 'direct' and 'indirect' duties in the old Kantian sense (see Sect. 3.1). This is not a distinction based on whom we have the duty *towards*, as the distinction is used in contemporary animal ethics. Rather, 'direct' duties are true duties, while 'indirect' duties are accidental means for fulfilling duty (see Timmermann 2005b, 140). For example, to be beneficent is a true or 'direct' duty, but to use our own sympathetic feelings as a catalyst for moral action is an indirect duty (MM 6:456.25).

Among duties to others, Kant distinguishes between duties of love and duties of respect. The former ask us to be beneficent, grateful, and sympathetic towards others—stances appropriate to the promotion of their happiness. The latter ask us to recognise and act in accordance with the equal humanity of others. This requires that we refrain from being arrogant, from backbiting and ridicule, and in general from stances that view others as less in status as a being capable of morality. This even requires that we put an upper limit to our beneficence, since at some point overbearing beneficence becomes condescending. Kantianism for Animals endorses a version of this view:

Practical love and non-exaltation

We ought to reconcile practical love for animals with a maxim of non-exaltation.

Practical love comprises the ends and activities we pursue in order to promote the happiness of others. Here, Kantianism for Animals stays fairly close to Kant. To repeat, the kind of 'happiness' the framework asks us to promote is hedonic in nature. It is a matter of feeling good. However, practical love also requires us to recognise that others are agents who are able to pursue and produce their own happiness. They may do so by means of instrumental practical reason, consciously picking means they deem appropriate to the end of happiness. Alternatively, there may be evolved patterns of action that produce happiness or some of its prerequisites, like health and flourishing. So what we should do, more often than not, is to help along others' self-chosen endeavours—so long as they still plausibly promote their happiness.

However, Kantianism for Animals does not endorse Kant's conception of 'duties of respect' exactly as he presents it. What Kant considers a 'duty of respect to others', Kantianism for Animals considers a duty of non-exaltation *to self, merely regarding others*. We do have a duty not to 'exalt' ourselves above others along the lines suggested by Kant. But this duty derives from the end of our own moral perfection, which requires that we recognise, and act in accordance with, our own moral capacities. We should neither lower ourselves below the status of a being capable of goodness, nor exaggerate our own moral worth (and relatedly, our worthiness of happiness). When it comes to other autonomous human beings, we should regard them as equals sharing our fundamental moral predicament, the struggle between inclination and duty. When it comes to nonautonomous animals, we should regard them as morally incomparable to us, as neither more nor less deserving of their happiness. We exalt ourselves above animals by being arrogant and viewing ourselves as categorically elevated above them in virtue of our moral capacities, but also by being beneficent from an insufficiently humble mindset.

Another noteworthy aspect of Kantianism for Animals is that according to this framework, reason and feelings each play an indispensable part in moral life. Rational beings autonomously impose the moral law on themselves by means of reason, and actions never get their moral worth from the feelings that have helped cause them. But the fulfilment of our duties towards others is always accompanied by certain feelings about them, ourselves, and the moral law. Hence, Kantianism for Animals does not parrot the rhetoric of reason found in many early works of animal ethics. Singer and Regan in particular insist that their moral concern for animals has its origins in reason, not in any feelings whatsoever (Regan 2004, xli–xliii; Singer 2002, xxif.). For both Singer (2002, xxi) and Regan (2004, lii), as well as for many non-philosophers in the animal rights movement (Groves 2001), this appeal to reason in contrast to emotion is a deliberate rhetorical tactic used to avoid being stereotyped as irrational. In any case, Kantianism for Animals does not need to rely on this tactic.

7.5   Motives Matter

One of Kant's most iconic claims in moral philosophy is that an action can only have moral worth if it springs from the right incentive, namely respect for the moral law. An action which is merely *in accordance* with duty may be permissible, but if its incentive is inclination, the action fails to have *moral worth*. Kantianism for Animals does not disagree with any of these parts of Kant's thought. It bears repeating, however, that incentives are not Kant's main unit of *moral guidance*—the obligatory ends are. For this reason, the recurrent allegation is false that Kant's singular—and patently unhelpful—piece of moral guidance is that we must act from duty. What is true, however, is that Kant's moral philosophy allots an important role to the things we may call the 'motives' of actions—the ends towards which they are directed, the maxims from which the actions spring, and the incentives that drive them:

Motives matter

Ends, maxims, and incentives matter for moral worth.

Of course, other views in animal ethics may agree with the above claim. Any sensible approach to animal ethics would consider actions wrong if they pursue cruelty as an end, for instance. However, Kantianism for Animals differs from influential views in its order of explanation. For Singer and Regan, to name prominent examples, what makes it wrong to pursue a cruel end is that it leads to bad outward acts—a failure to maximise utility or a violation of rights, respectively. For Kant, the *ethical* issue lies with the motives of actions in themselves, and outward acts are *ethically* wrong if they are connected to certain motives contrary to duty.

To sum up, I have used this intermission to capture the main features of Kantianism for Animals in five key claims. Kantianism for Animals distinctively claims the autonomously imposed moral law to be the normative basis of our duties towards animals. It claims that duties have explanatory, epistemic, and normative primacy over rights and claims. It adheres to a doctrine of obligatory ends according to which we have a duty to promote the happiness of others and a duty to pursue our own moral self-perfection. It claims that we must find the right balance between beneficence and non-exaltation vis à vis others. And it claims that our moral worth depends on the motives of actions broadly construed—the ends we set, the maxims from which our actions spring, and the incentives from which we act. Taken individually, not all of these five claims are novelties in the literature. But taken together, they characterise Kantianism for Animals as a novel and distinctive framework in animal ethics.

References

Benton, Ted. 1996. Animal rights. An eco-socialist view. In *Animal Rights. The Changing Debate*, ed. Robert Garner, 19–41. New York: New York University Press.

Diamond, Cora. 1978. Eating meat and eating people. *Philosophy* 53: 465–479.

Godfrey-Smith, Peter. 2021. Philosophers and other animals. *Aeon.*

Groves, Julian M. 2001. Animal rights and the politics of emotion: Folk constructions of emotion in the animal rights movement. In *Passionate politics: Emotions and social movements*, ed. Jeff Goodwin, James M. Jasper, and Francesca Polletta, 212–232. Chicago: University of Chicago Press.

Gruen, Lori. 2015. *Entangled empathy: An alternative ethic for our relationships with animals.* New York: Lantern Books.

Mohr, Georg. 2010. Moralische Rechte gibt es nicht. In *Recht und Moral*, ed. Hans Jörg Sandkühler, 63–80. Hamburg: Felix Meiner.

Narveson, Jan. 1987a. A case against animal rights. In *Advances in animal welfare science 1986/87*, ed. Michael W. Fox and Linda D. Mickley, 191–204. Dordrecht: Springer.

Narveson, Jan. 1987b. On a case for animal rights. *The Monist* 70: 31–49.

Regan, Tom. 2003. *Animal rights, human wrongs: An introduction to moral philosophy.* Lanham, MD: Rowman & Littlefield.

Regan, Tom. 2004. *The case for animal rights.* Berkeley/Los Angeles: University of California Press.

Singer, Peter. 2002. *Animal liberation.* New York: Ecco Press.

Timmermann, Jens. 2005a. Why Kant could not have been a utilitarian. *Utilitas* 17: 243–264.

Timmermann, Jens. 2005b. When the tail wags the dog: Animal welfare and indirect duty in Kantian ethics. *Kantian Review* 10: 127–149.

Timmermann, Jens. 2015. What's wrong with "deontology"? *Proceedings of the Aristotelian Society* 115: 75–92.

Wood, Allen W. 2007. *Kantian ethics.* Cambridge: Cambridge University Press.

PART III

Using the Framework

CHAPTER 8

A Kantian Argument Against Using Animals

8.1 'External' Arguments Against Using Animals

So far in this book, I have proposed amendments to Kant's moral philosophy that enable us to include animals in moral concern. Precisely those who are typically inclined to dismiss Kant's philosophy due to its disagreeable consequences in animal ethics thus receive new theoretical resources. In this final part of the book, my aim is to illustrate what animal ethicists might do with these resources. The arguments in this chapter and the subsequent two are not, strictly speaking, 'implications' or 'applications' of the proposed theory. The coming chapters are going to take the perspective of Kantianism for Animals as a starting point, but will each make some additional philosophical move or add a further modification of the framework. In doing so, they rather present creative variations over themes from the book up to this point. My hope in presenting these variations is that they encourage other animal ethicists to come up with ideas of their own for how to use or amend the framework.

To start with, one striking feature that sets Kantianism for Animals apart from many other views in animal ethics is its characteristic emphasis on the motive of action. Not only does this framework put great weight on what Kant calls the *incentive* of an action (either respect for the moral law or inclination), but its material moral guidance comes primarily in the unit of *duties of virtue*, which name the *ends* for which we ought to strive and the *practical-emotional stances* which we ought to adopt. This can

© The Author(s) 2022
N. D. Müller, *Kantianism for Animals*, The Palgrave Macmillan
Animal Ethics Series,
https://doi.org/10.1007/978-3-031-01930-2_8

come in handy for animal ethicists when more traditional considerations—
say, about the wrongness of incurring bad *consequences* for animals—fail to
adequately express what is ethically problematic about a practice.

One of the most prominent examples is the practice of *animal use.*
What is at issue here is the use of *live* animals as means to human ends, be
it in food industries, in research, in entertainment, and so on.[1] In the animal rights movement and in academic animal ethics, there exists a camp of
people who think that there is something *inherently* objectionable about
using animals as means to our happiness. A view along these lines often
underpins veganism. However, it is surprisingly difficult to find a direct
argument for this view in the literature. I am going to argue that Kantianism
for Animals offers a novel argument against most of what we ordinarily call
'animal use'. In doing so, my approach adds to the traditional case against
animal use, while also helping to *specify* what makes animal use problematic.

My argument will take the following steps. First, I will explain in more
detail what gaps there are to fill in the traditional case against animal use.
Secondly, I will explain what Kantianism for Animals can contribute. The
argument, in a nutshell, will be that what critics mean by 'animal use' is
the treatment of animals as a means to the end of our own happiness. The
trouble with the associated stance towards others is that it treats our own
self-interest as a *limiting condition* on our duty to promote the happiness
of others. But our duties should restrict our pursuit of self-interest, not
vice versa. This stance, I will suggest, is opposed to duty in a similar way
as the vices discussed by Kant in the *Doctrine of Virtue.* Therefore, animal
use is opposed to duty. I conclude by highlighting some features which set
this Kantian argument apart from earlier arguments.

To situate the argument in the literature, consider the traditional dialectic when it comes to the ethics of animal use: In one camp, there are
said to be the moderates, dubbed 'welfarists'. On their view, the strategic
focus of the animal rights movement should lie on gradually improving
the conditions under which animals are used. In the other camp, there are
the radicals, usually designated as 'abolitionists'. Rather than merely
demanding improved conditions for animals, abolitionists are understood
to demand the total and sudden abolition of all animal use (Francione
1996; Dunayer 2004; Francione and Garner 2010; Wrenn 2012).

---

[1] Of course, the *dead bodies* of animals are also used as means to human ends. I return to
the use of dead animal bodies in Chap. 9.

A note on the terminology: The notion of 'abolitionism' and the associated abolitionism-welfarism distinction are problematic for several reasons.[2] First, the term 'abolitionism' is purposely taken from the history of American slavery (e.g. Francione 1996, 47). The practice of drawing comparisons between animal exploitation and the enslavement of human beings has been subject to strong criticism (Kim 2018). Secondly, the abolitionism-welfarism distinction presents a false dichotomy. One might also set out to abolish all animal use *gradually*, by means of incremental improvements in welfare regulation (Francione and Garner 2010, 135). Hence, the distinction is not exhaustive, although it misleadingly appears so.[3] Third, the abolitionism-welfarism distinction equates incrementalism with incrementalism regarding *animal welfare improvements*. But one could just as well be an incrementalist in other respects. For instance, one might try to abolish animal use by incrementally changing animals' legal status as property, granting them more and more features of legal subjecthood. This trend of 'subjectivisation' is already visible in certain legislations (Stucki 2016, 138, see Sect. 1.1). One might also pursue a strategy of small steps to reduce subsidies to animal industries and to increase people's ability to leave these industries, but the abolitionism-welfarism distinction obscures these options. To avoid all these difficulties, I will refrain from using the label 'abolitionism' altogether. Instead of arguments 'for abolitionism', I will simply be talking about arguments 'against animal use'.

It can be useful to distinguish between two types of arguments against animal use: *Internal* arguments scrutinise the notion of 'animal use' and provide an explanation why all animal use is inherently objectionable. *External* arguments, by contrast, merely point out objectionable *consequences* or *preconditions* of animal use. For instance, an animal advocate might explain that suffering and death are routinely inflicted upon animals in all industries that use them. An external argument then implies that ending all animal use is the only surefire way to avoid bad consequences, or that the avoidance of bad prerequisites also entails the end of animal use.

External arguments can have certain practical advantages. Elaborating on the various respects in which animal use leads to suffering and death can be a powerful rhetorical device. It also gives animal advocates a

---

[2] For an overview of criticisms, see Wrenn (2012). Here, I merely mention the three issues which motivate me to refrain from using the term 'abolitionism'.

[3] This position is standardly called 'new welfarism' (Francione 1998, 45).

welcome opportunity to educate their audience on the grim reality of animal use. A weakness of such arguments is however that they cannot determine whether there is anything *inherently* wrong with animal use. Hence, the most natural response to external arguments speaks out in favour of more 'humane' animal use. After all, if bad consequences are all that is problematic about animal use, then the parsimonious solution lies in adopting or developing practices of animal use that avoid these consequences. However, animal advocates who argue against animal use are typically not interested in this search for 'humane' animal use. Their gut feeling tells them rather that there is something morally awry with wanting to 'use' animals in the first place. External arguments fail to capture and convey this feeling. So external arguments can steer the discussion in a direction unwelcome to the radicals who have started the conversation in the first place, and they fail to capture the point that motivates them. For this reason, radical animal advocates should not content themselves with *only* external arguments against animal use.

Internal arguments against animal use are not completely absent from the debate. Torres hints at one when he writes: "The moment we use another being instrumentally, as means to our ends, we have denied that being its right to exist on its own terms, whether that being is human or non-human" (Torres 2007, 26).[4] However, such remarks can usually be found in the margins of animal advocates' texts, while the main body relies on external arguments. This is certainly true for the work of the two scholars most commonly associated with the label 'abolitionism': Regan, and the label's inventor, Francione. Let me briefly explain why their arguments against using animals should be considered external.

As Regan's readers might expect, he takes issue with any treatment of animals which violates their *rights*. He makes this point explicit when it comes to animal agriculture:

> It is true—and this point bears emphasis—that *the ultimate objective of the rights view is the total dissolution of the animal industry as we know it*, an objective that should hardly be surprising, given the rights view's verdict that, as presently conducted, this industry violates the rights of farm animals. (Regan 2004, 348)

---

[4] As an aside, this claim is overstated. We treat postal workers as means to the end of getting our mail delivered, but we do not deny them any right to exist on their own terms. Of course, Torres is getting at another kind of instrumental attitude towards others. My point is that he does not precisely nail down this more exploitative instrumental attitude.

Regan also favours the dissolution of other branches of animal use, such as in biomedical research (Regan 2004, 388), education (Regan 2004, 364), and hunting and trapping (Regan 2004, 353). In general, the rights view "calls on each of us to strive to make the world better by withholding our direct support from the major animal exploiting industries" (Regan 2003, 118).

It is fairly obvious how the *actual* ways in which animals are used violate the central right postulated by Regan, namely the right not to be harmed (Regan 2004, 279ff.). This is so especially if we consider death to be a harm, as Regan does (Regan 2004, 99ff.). Most actual instances of animal use, including in the egg and dairy industry, require the killing of surplus or unprofitable animals, and great bodily and psychological harm is inflicted on the respective animals for human gain. Hence, the most straightforward general argument against animal use we can draw from Regan's rights view runs as follows:

Regan's argument against animal use

(1) Using animals leads to violations of the right not to be harmed.
(2) It is objectionable to violate the right not to be harmed.
(3) Therefore, using animals is objectionable.

But notice that this is an external argument. It moves from a claim about an objectionable consequence of animal use (1) to the wrongness of animal use (3). But first, one could question if (1) is true without exception, or whether a harmless mode of animal use is possible. Secondly, even harmful animal use does not consist *only* of harmful actions. What the argument primarily shows, then, is that *certain actions* in the context of use are objectionable, namely those that inflict suffering and death on animals. In animal agriculture, for instance, animal use also involves feeding animals, cleaning their enclosures, providing some medical care, and so on. Is the only problem with using animals that it (usually) ends up involving certain objectionable actions, or does Regan also have something more direct to say against animal use *as such*?

The general difficulty in constructing an internal argument from Regan's approach is that the 'rights view' is, fundamentally, a theory of moral boundaries that we must not transgress. Rights are "a kind of protective moral shield, something we might picture as an invisible No Trespassing sign" (Regan 2003, 25). Hence, the rights theorist criticises actions in terms of their consequences on rights-bearers, not in terms of the practices or motives of the trespasser. But this makes it very hard to make a case without loopholes against any particular practice, unless rights-violating consequences form a part of its definition.

When it comes to the practice of animal use, the straightforward work-around for the rights theorist would be to posit a blanket *right not to be used*. No such right appears in Regan's work. The closest, it seems, is the right to respectful treatment (Regan 2004, 276). To make the case against animal use, we would have to appeal to an account of what constitutes respectful treatment and to the premiss that there is something disrespectful about using animals *per se*. This does not sound too far off Regan's views. But what is it to treat someone with respect, Regan-style? As he puts it himself, the 'respect principle' demands that we do not treat individuals "*as if their value depended upon their utility* relative to the interests of others" (Regan 2004, 248f.). To be sure, this description fits most actual instances of animal use. When animals are routinely killed, packed, and sold, this treatment indeed looks as if it is guided by purely instrumental considerations. But again, is it so clear that using animals *entails* that we treat them as merely instrumentally valuable? Might we not also, in using animals, treat them as *both* inherently *and* instrumentally valuable, or switch between the two modes of treatment during the process of animal use?

Here, the undesirable effect of external arguments begins to set in. The debate from this point onwards revolves around examples of supposedly 'humane' animal use. It would frankly seem ad hoc for Regan to argue that an instance of animal use which does not violate *any* other rights, including the right not to be harmed, still violates the right to respectful treatment. In other words, the only uncontroversial examples of violations of the right to respectful treatment also involve, at the same time, violations of other rights. Factory farming is clearly in violation of the right to respectful treatment, but only because it also violates the right not to be harmed. But then, Regan's approach leaves it open whether there is anything morally objectionable about animal use as such. There is no internal argument against animal use to be found here, only an argument against typical rights-violating consequences of animal use.

We encounter the inverse problem when reading Francione: Where Regan's argument mainly revolves around the *consequences* of animal use, Francione's revolves around a *prerequisite* of animal use, namely the legal status of animals as property:

The abolition of animal exploitation necessarily requires a paradigm shift away from the status of animals as property [...]. Personhood is inconsistent with the property status of animals and with any animal use, however 'humane'. (Francione and Garner 2010, 4)

Francione's main line of reasoning is that animals' legal status as property puts them on unequal legal footing with persons (Francione 1995, 18f.). After all, the interests of legal persons can enjoy the special protection granted by legal rights, the interests of property cannot (Francione 1995, 32). Therefore, even trivial interests of human beings and corporations can legally trump the most vital interests of animals. To pick an example, this inequality is what accounts for the legality of killing animals merely for monetary gain (ibid.). The interest in killing animals may be covered by a legal right protecting economic liberty, say, while the animal lacks any legal rights whatsoever which could protect its interest in not being killed. It is clear which side the law must favour. In order to solve the problem once and for all, Francione calls for the abolishment of animals' property status. That *animal use* must be abolished is then merely a corollary. To roughly summarise:

Francione's argument against animal use

(4) Using animals requires treating them as property.
(5) Treating animals as property is objectionable.
(6) Therefore, using animals is objectionable.

This is an external argument in that it moves from a premiss about an objectionable prerequisite of animal use (4) to the wrongness of animal use (6). Against the backdrop of his argument, Francione's primary interlocutor is 'welfarism'. If we merely aim to improve the conditions under which animals are used, argues Francione, we fail to address the real problem. In this context, the claim that *all* animal use is objectionable does not take centre stage. And indeed, it is rather unclear why Francione's argument against the property status of animals would be an argument against all animal use as such. It only clearly condemns animal use that relies on animals' property status. The argument is not designed to cover, say, instances of animal use that occur outside of any organised polity, or in a polity that does not recognise the institution of property. And even if we take the institution of property for granted, the question remains why we could not *both* furnish animals with legal rights *and* simultaneously continue to use them, assuming this use does not violate their rights (as Cochrane suggests, Cochrane 2012).

The situation is similar in the work of other writers who oppose animal use, such as Dunayer (2004), Torres (2007), and Wrenn (2015). Because the typical consequences (and arguably, the prerequisites) of animal use are so obviously morally objectionable, opponents of animal use have not focused on showing that animal use is *inherently* objectionable. But for this reason, animal ethics has yet to see an internal argument against animal use. So the case against animal use is still missing the crucial piece that really makes it tick. In the following, let me explain how Kantianism for Animals can help to fill this gap.

8.2   A Kantian-for-Animals 'Internal' Argument Against Animal Use

As we have seen in Chaps. 2 and 7, Kant devotes much of his attention in ethics to duties in terms of *practical-emotional stances* which we ought either to adopt or avoid. Those we ought to adopt are simply called *duties of virtue*, and they name practical-emotional stances which befit our moral task: to promote the happiness of others and our own moral perfection. The stances we ought to avoid Kant calls *vices* (MM 6:458.21; MM 6:465.04). They are attitudes or mindsets we adopt voluntarily which are "directly (*contrarie*) opposed" (MM 6:458.20) to duty. That is not to say that vices make it strictly impossible for us to act as we ought. But they are unhelpful for our moral task, so that even if we do manage to act as we ought, it was only *despite* our vices. Insofar as Kant morally discourages vices, he views adopting them and acting from them as ethically objectionable.

To name an example, consider Kant's prohibition of *malicious glee*. By this term, Kant means a practical-emotional stance we adopt whenever we take pleasure in the misfortune of others (MM 6:459.36). Evidently, this is a morally dubious stance, given the basic predicament of the Kantian moral agent: to strive for the pleasant by nature while striving for the good by reason. If our duty is to promote the happiness of others, of course we should not set out to take pleasure in their misfortune. The stance of malicious glee is a stance directly opposed to duty. Therefore, it is a vice, and it is objectionable to adopt it, let alone act from it.

Kantianism for Animals offers a novel objection against animal use: What we usually mean by 'animal use' is a practice inherently based on a stance that is a Kantian vice. To back up this claim with an argument, let me give an account of what stance I presume to be inherent in animal use and an explanation why it is contrary to duty.

First, what stance should we presume an animal user to take towards animals? The easiest option would be to adapt Regan's account of disrespect and claim that animal users take a *purely instrumental* stance towards animals, viewing them not as patients whose happiness is to be promoted, but purely as ordinary things to be used to our benefit. It would be straightforward that such a stance would be opposed to duty, hence a vice. However, as we have already seen, it is uncharitable to suppose that all animal users are quite so cold-hearted. Someone might use animals while viewing them as simultaneously inherently valuable *and* instrumentally valuable, or switch between the two perspectives from one moment to the next.

More plausible and charitable is it to suppose that animal users act from a mindset that contains at least an element of practical benevolence: The animal user sets out to promote the happiness of the animal *insofar as it is compatible* with a certain human end. An animal user who acts from this stance is not bound to promote the happiness of animals only insofar as it *contributes* to a further end (say, feeding animals to fatten them up). They may also take deliberate steps to promote the happiness of animals in ways that do not recognisably affect the further end (say, petting the animals to comfort them). As for the further end involved, we need not be overly specific. One might use animals in order to create some product, render some service, or simply to make a living. Inherent in the notion of 'animal use'—the thing opponents of animal use are against—is however that it is a practice we pursue *for our own sake* at the end of the day. It is a practice devised to promote an end the animal user pursues for the sake of their own happiness. So we can characterise the stance inherent in practices of animal use as putting a self-interested limit on practical benevolence.

Secondly, why is such a stance a Kantian vice? To be sure, putting a self-interested limit on practical benevolence is not as simple a vice as malicious glee. It does not straightforwardly associate another's misfortune with pleasure, and the moral challenge it poses is not that it makes us squarely antagonistic towards others. Rather, putting such a limit on practical benevolence is opposed to duty because it presents our own, non-moral ends as superior to the obligatory ends of pure reason. It puts a structural obstacle in the way of our pursuit of the obligatory end of another's happiness. Our pursuit of this obligatory end should not be restricted by any non-moral ends, but only by our other duties.

As we saw in Sect. 2.4 above, the vocabulary of practical-emotional stances represents a middle level of generality at which we can describe our duties. At a higher level of generality, our duties can be put in terms of the two obligatory ends, which are the happiness of others and our own moral perfection. Conversely, zooming in on our ethical duties towards others, we can also describe them in a more fine-grained way, in terms of the ends of others we ought to adopt. An important point, recall, is that Kant does not ask us to simply adopt another's *next best* end. Our duty is rather to assist others in their own endeavours, insofar as those endeavours in turn promote their happiness. If we help along another's own endeavours in a way that ultimately *undermines* their happiness instead of promoting it, we have not been beneficent. But this is what we do in the seemingly more beneficent actions involved in animal use—say, when we feed an animal, but only in order to fatten it up for slaughter. By providing food, we may help along the animal's next best end, namely food intake, but we do not promote the *point* of this end which would connect it to the animal's happiness, namely nutrition and ultimately survival.[5] So according to a Kantian conception of practical benevolence, the actions an animal user takes to promote the animal's happiness 'locally', but without regard for its happiness 'globally', do not qualify as truly benevolent.

Returning to the vocabulary of practical-emotional stances, Kantianism for Animals' basic argument against animal use runs as follows:

The Kantian internal argument against animal use

(7) To 'use' animals is to put a self-interested limit on practical benevolence towards them.

(8) Putting a self-interested limit on practical benevolence towards others is a vice.

(9) Therefore, the animal user's stance is a vice.

It may be somewhat surprising to see a Kantian argument against animal use which does *not* appeal to the principle that others must not be

---

[5] The 'point' here is a matter of biological functionality. For a fuller account why biological functionality matters in Kantianism for Animals, see Sect. 6.4.

treated as mere means. As we have seen in Chap. 4, Kantianism for Animals relies on a reading of Kantian ethics on which the Formula of Humanity—which asks us never to treat humanity in our own person or in the person of any other as a mere means (GMS 4:429.10–13)—does not play a central role in the derivation of specific duties. It is a purely formal principle of autonomous willing which tells us something about *how* a good will wills, without giving us a very clear picture of *what* it wills. If a Kantian argument instead started with the premiss that animals must never be treated as mere means, the obvious question would be what 'treatment as mere means' denotes. Although one could of course have myriad different interpretations, and each might make for an interesting argument against animal use, I want to suggest that premiss (8) offers a prima facie plausible analysis: We 'treat animals as mere means' whenever we treat any of our own non-moral ends as a limiting condition on the promotion of the happiness of animals. Understood thus, the internal Kantian argument *does* ask us not to treat animals as mere means, without however putting any weight on this obscure formulation.

The most straightforward objection to the Kantian internal argument is that it condemns too much. It may appear to condemn all treatment of animals as means. But this is not true. What the argument condemns, per premiss (8), is treating our own non-moral ends as limiting conditions on the obligatory ends—treating them as *mere* means, on a certain understanding of the term. As long as we regard the obligatory ends as superior to our non-moral ends, however, there is nothing inherently vicious about our treatment of others as means. In this case, we are treating others as means without treating them as *mere* means.

This however leads to another objection to the argument: We can also use animals for *moral* ends rather than non-moral ones. For instance, one might argue that animal users have a duty to promote the happiness of their own family members, and making a living using animals can promote this end. Or, alternatively, one could say that animal users might use animals minimally, merely for their own sustenance which they have an indirect ethical duty to self to secure. In either case, the animal user is not guilty of putting a self-interested limit on their practical benevolence. Their benevolence would be restricted by other duties only. Hence, the argument does not condemn them. So the argument fails to condemn all animal use for human gain.

This objection merits a three-part response: First, we should not be too quick to grant that actual animal users are guided by moral ends. If all they wanted was to promote the happiness of others, but the happiness of their family members happened to be at odds with the happiness of animals, this would represent an apparent conflict of duties. But then, we should expect agents to respond to the situation as an apparent moral conflict: They should feel *pro tanto* regret, they should search for a third option that violates neither duty, and they should make a serious effort to avoid encountering the same apparent conflict of duties again in the future. Animal users who fit this description, and only they, are let off the hook by the Kantian argument. People who use animals in a self-righteous and routine way are not.

Secondly, if the agent does sincerely take herself to be caught in a moral conflict, there remains the question why she takes the animals to draw the short straw. Why does the promotion of the happiness of certain human beings trump the promotion of the happiness of these animals? If the response relies on any claim to the effect that human beings are more valuable, more deserving of their happiness than animals, endorsing it runs counter to the duty of non-exaltation. Animals are neither more nor less deserving of their happiness than human beings, since they do not stand under the moral law in the first place.

Thirdly, if the agent does have a good reason to prioritise the happiness of specific human beings (or other animals) over the happiness of specific animals—that is, a reason which we can adopt without violating the duty of non-exaltation above others—then the Kantian argument may indeed let the agent off the hook. However, I would suggest that using animals as means to *moral* ends, under such circumstances, is simply not the practice of 'animal use' to which radical animal advocates are opposed. What they mean by 'animal use' is using animals somewhat deliberately, as contingent means to the end of our own happiness, treating our own non-moral ends as a limiting condition on the obligatory end of another's happiness. The critique of animal use as a Kantian vice captures this.

Before I conclude, let me highlight some noteworthy aspects of the Kantian argument against animal use. First, the argument implies that even seemingly beneficent actions towards animals—feeding them, cleaning their enclosure, providing them with medical care, and so on—fail to have moral worth if they occur within the context of animal use, and are even objectionable, since acting on a vice is objectionable even if the consequences happen to be morally desirable. External arguments would suggest that such actions make animal use at least marginally better. Hence, they tend to provoke a response in terms of gradual improvements to animal welfare. Kantianism for Animals rejects this response from the start, since what it primarily condemns is the *stance* inherent in animal use, no matter how 'humane' that use ends up being. Of course, we should think twice before taking the Kantian argument as a basis for policy decisions or political strategy. As we saw in Chap. 1, a Kantian *ethic* fundamentally addresses the question how we should want to act, not what is politically or legally legitimate, let alone what is strategically advisable. So what the argument shows is not that all animal use can or should be immediately prohibited, but only that there are reasons for individuals to find the practice morally repugnant.

Secondly, however, the Kantian internal argument's premises imply more than just a duty of *abstinence*. The argument presupposes a demanding, even ambitious account of our duties towards animals, which asks us to promote the happiness of animals (and human beings). As long as the actual systems of animal use are as harmful to animals (and human beings) as they are today, we should actively oppose these systems for the sake of our duties to others.

Third, I should point out that there might be cases of apparent 'animal use' which are not condemned even by the internal argument, due to the fuzziness of the notion. For instance, we might *derive utility* from animals without putting human aims first. One variant of this is somewhat coincidental or non-institutionalised utility derived from animals. A horse may pass by your garden and leave some droppings. If you collect these droppings to fertilise your roses, the internal argument does not condemn you, if you did not treat your own ends as a limiting condition on the promotion of the happiness of animals. But presumably, the philosophers and animal activists who oppose animal use in general would not condemn you either. Another variant is animal use that is in the service of the animals themselves. If a not-for-profit farm animal sanctuary offers guided tours to visitors to help raise funds, one might claim this constitutes a borderline case of 'using' the animals for fundraising and educational purposes. But here, the human end of raising funds for the sanctuary might just be the best means to the end of the animals' happiness, and not a limiting condition. The internal argument either does not condemn this, or even encourages it (assuming, of course, that there is no better way of raising funds).

This is effectively an animal-friendly variant of the 'moral ends' argument discussed earlier. Again, using animals as means to strictly moral ends, especially if that moral end is the best possible promotion of their own happiness, is not the practice of 'animal use' that is at issue in the debate.

Let me also emphasise some conclusions that do *not* follow from this chapter's argument. First, it is sometimes suggested that an end to animal use would necessarily require the cessation of any and all *interactions* with animals. Thus, Korsgaard claims that 'abolitionism' is based on the view that all our interactions with others must be based on consent, but animals cannot consent, therefore we must not interact with animals at all (Korsgaard 2018, 177f.). In a similar vein, Donaldson and Kymlicka say of the 'abolitionist' camp: "The bottom line is that we must end all human use of, *and interaction with*, domesticated animals" (Donaldson and Kymlicka 2011, 78, emphasis added). But no such thing follows from the argument in this chapter. What the argument condemns is not interacting with animals, but interacting with them in a way that treats our own non-moral ends as a limiting condition on our promotion of their happiness. In fact, refusing to interact with animals altogether would be inherently detrimental to the promotion of their happiness just as much as 'using' animals is.

Secondly, the argument also does not imply that animals ought to be 'liberated' from human interaction in a way that is insensitive to their interests—a supposed demand of the 'abolitionist' camp against which Cochrane takes great care to argue (Cochrane 2012, 7). What the Kantian argument in this chapter does imply, however, is that more is to be said against animal use than just that it violates the interests of animals (whether these interests be protected by rights or not). The argument at issue is distinctively ethical in that it concerns the configuration of motives that determine the moral agent's actions. Hence, Kantianism for Animals can be a helpful complement to an interest-based theory of rights. While a theory of rights sets up certain moral boundaries for our self-interested treatment of animals, Kantianism for Animals criticises the very way in which our treatment of animals is self-interested.

Let me summarise. I have argued that animal ethics has not yet seen an internal argument against animal use. An internal argument, as opposed to an external one, is not so much concerned with consequences or prerequisites of animal use. Rather it aims to scrutinise the notion of 'animal use' itself and point out an objectionable element. To use animals, I have proposed, is to use them as means to the end of our own happiness. When we use animals, we do *not* necessarily treat them in a purely instrumental way, denying altogether that we have duties towards them. Rather, we should understand animal users to take a stance which puts a self-interested limit on their practical benevolence towards others. The trouble with this stance is that it treats our non-moral ends (our own happiness) as a limiting condition on the obligatory end of another's happiness. This restriction is opposed to duty, and the resulting practical benevolence is not the kind of practical benevolence duty demands. Hence, the animal user's stance is a Kantian vice.

REFERENCES

Cochrane, Alasdair. 2012. *Animal rights without liberation: Applied ethics and human obligations.* New York: Columbia University Press.

Donaldson, Sue, and Will Kymlicka. 2011. *Zoopolis: A political theory of animal rights.* New York: Oxford University Press.

Dunayer, Joan. 2004. *Speciesism.* Derwood, MD: Ryce Publishing.

Francione, Gary L. 1995. *Animals, property, and the law.* Philadelphia: Temple University Press.

Francione, Gary L. 1996. *Rain without thunder: The ideology of the animal rights movement.* Philadelphia: Temple University Press.

Francione, Gary L. 1998. Animal rights movement and new welfarism. In *Encyclopedia of animal rights and animal welfare,* ed. Marc Bekoff and Carron A. Meaney, 45. London: Fitzroy Dearborn Publishers.

Francione, Gary L., and Robert Garner. 2010. *The animal rights debate: Abolition or regulation?* New York: Columbia University Press.

Kim, Claire J. 2018. Abolition. In *Critical terms for animal studies,* ed. Lori Gruen, 15–32. Chicago: University of Chicago Press.

Korsgaard, Christine M. 2018. *Fellow creatures: Our obligations to the other animals.* Oxford: Oxford University Press.

Regan, Tom. 2003. Animal rights, human wrongs: An introduction to moral philosophy. Lanham, MD: Rowman & Littlefield.

Regan, Tom. 2004. *The case for animal rights.* Berkeley/Los Angeles: University of California Press.

Stucki, Saskia. 2016. Grundrechte für Tiere: Eine Kritik des geltenden Tierschutzrechts und rechtstheoretische Grundlegung von Tierrechten im Rahmen einer Neupositionierung des Tieres als Rechtssubjekt. Baden-Baden: Nomos.

Torres, Bob. 2007. *Making a killing: The political economy of animal rights.* Oakland/Edinburgh/West Virginia: AK Press.

Wrenn, Corey L. 2012. Abolitionist animal rights: Critical comparisons and challenges within the animal rights movement. *Interface* 4: 438–458.

Wrenn, Corey L. 2015. *A rational approach to animal rights.* New York: Palgrave Macmillan.

CHAPTER 9

A Kantian Argument Against Eating Animals

9.1 The Philosophical Stalemate Regarding Vegetarianism

We have just seen that the idea of a duty of virtue—a duty to adopt a certain end or practical-emotional stance—can make Kantianism for Animals a helpful resource for animal ethicists. Another noteworthy feature of the framework is its recognition of duties *towards self*, duties which aim at moral self-perfection. Now, this book started with the insight that these duties *alone* cannot provide an adequate account of our moral relations to animals (see Chap. 3). However, once we recognise duties to animals, the notion of a duty to self can be a helpful addition to the animal ethical vocabulary. In particular, Kantianism for Animals opens up the option that there are certain duties towards self which only exist *because* we have duties towards animals. Appealing to such duties can be useful when we try to express, for example, what is problematic about certain ways of treating animals that do not directly *harm* them.

I would like to discuss the most prominent instance of such treatment in this chapter: eating dead animals. Influential arguments against eating animals in the literature have focused on the wrongness of inflicting suffering and death. These arguments are primarily directed against *slaughtering* animals, not strictly against *eating* them once they are dead. In Diamond's words, "there is nothing in the discussion which suggests that a cow is *not* something to eat; it is only that one must not help the process

© The Author(s) 2022
N. D. Müller, *Kantianism for Animals*, The Palgrave Macmillan
Animal Ethics Series,
https://doi.org/10.1007/978-3-031-01930-2_9

along" (Diamond 1978, 468). Subsequently, various philosophers have tried to show that the wrongness of eating animals can be derived from the wrongness of killing them. But these arguments are fraught with serious difficulties.

My aim in this chapter is to show how Kantianism for Animals can capture and convey the moral outlook of those vegetarians who refuse to see animals as 'something to eat'. I will argue that ordinary meat eating exhibits a certain thoughtlessness or inconsideration towards animals which violates a duty towards self. In our treatment of dead bodies, we ought to cultivate a sense of the moral importance of others—that is, of the moral importance of those towards whom we used to have duties. By turning the dead into mundane resources, ordinary meat eating is contrary to this duty.

My discussion will take the following steps: First, I am going to briefly survey the most influential arguments in favour of vegetarianism. Secondly, I will lay out the additional resources Kantianism for Animals has to offer. It is only because we have duties towards animals, I argue, that we have a duty *towards self* to treat their deaths as morally important events, their bodies as morally important objects. The indifference with which ordinary meat eaters treat dead animal bodies then appears as a vice opposed to our duties to self. This also shows that vegetarianism can simultaneously be a matter of how we treat ourselves and how we treat animals.

Over twenty years ago, Curnutt declared that the philosophical debate about vegetarianism had reached a "stalemate" (Curnutt 1997, 153). By 'vegetarianism', he and I both mean the refusal, on moral grounds, to eat the body parts of animals who were once capable of happiness. Dominant approaches primarily view the practice of eating animals through the lens of *harm*—eating animals is objectionable due to its connection to the infliction of suffering and death. But such arguments evidently leave open the question whether there is anything morally repugnant about eating animals *in itself*.

Consider, for instance, the argument prominently featured in Singer's *Animal Liberation*. As one might expect, Singer is mainly concerned with the suffering inflicted in the meat industry: "It is not practically possible to rear animals for food on a large scale without inflicting considerable suffering" (Singer 2002, 160). This suffering is not outweighed by so much pleasure that the meat industry could pass as utility-maximising. Therefore, we ought to abolish the meat industry and not uphold it by buying and consuming meat.

Regan has objected to Singer's style of reasoning. As he puts it in *The Case for Animal Rights*:

> For the utilitarian [...] *it is an open question* whether the harm done to farm animals, even the harm they are made to bear in factory farms, is justifiable. *If* the aggregated consequences turn out to be optimal, *then* the harm is justified. (Regan 2004, 350)

The essential difference between Singer and Regan in this specific debate is that Singer still allows for a certain trade-off of human and animal interests, whereas Regan views this trading-off itself as morally repugnant if the rights of individuals are at stake (ibid.). In principle, it could have turned out that factory farming results in maximum utility, all things considered.[1] For Singer, this would imply that factory farming is morally desirable. For Regan, factory farming would still be unacceptable, since the rights of individuals must not be violated merely for the sake of greater overall utility. This disagreement about the permissibility of moral trade-offs however occurs against the backdrop of fundamental agreement that the wrongness of eating meat is a matter of the harm that is causally connected to it.

The merits of these arguments notwithstanding, they still view the morality of eating animals almost exclusively through the lens of suffering and death inflicted on animals who are, up until that point, alive. They are not so much concerned with the treatment of dead animals' bodies itself. And an argument of this type will inevitably leave open certain loopholes and grey areas. What about a case Diamond brings up, of a cow suddenly struck by lightning (Diamond 1978, 468)? No further harm follows causally from the act of eating this body. Still, many real-life vegetarians would presumably find something objectionable in treating the cow's dead body as just another foodstuff.

This problem extends beyond mere loopholes. Under real economic circumstances, the relation between individual meat consumption and the

---

[1] Hare has argued that a moderate version of animal agriculture results in maximum utility, since it enables many more animals to live that have at least a marginally pleasant life (Hare 1993). Once again (see Sect. 8.1), how we frame a moral problem determines which solutions seem the most parsimonious and straightforward. Singer's framing of the problem suggests that we should move towards a mode of animal agriculture that produces less suffering, as in Hare's vision. Regan's framing suggests that only food production without slaughter is acceptable.

infliction of suffering and death on animals is complicated (as Hudson has pointed out, Hudson 1993). Fischer helpfully summarises this 'causal impotence problem' in the following example:

> A grocery store can't get a single can of Spam from its warehouse; it has to request boxes or maybe entire pallets. The warehouse's supplier doesn't deliver individual boxes or pallets but only truckloads. And the supplier's supplier—which may not be the meat-packing plant itself, but let's suppose it is—has a strong incentive to produce as much as anyone might buy. (Fischer 2018, 244)

Under these circumstances, the individual consumer's choice to buy and consume meat has no direct and foreseeable consequence regarding the infliction of suffering and death on animals.

One solution to this problem is to appeal to collective responsibility: Though individual consumption makes little difference, collective consumption does. So we bear responsibility for the wrongs of the meat industry *as parts of the collectives to whose consumption the industry responds* (Hudson 1993). As Curnutt has pointed out, however, this argument counterintuitively assigns blame to individuals who could not have prevented the wrong (Curnutt 1997, 165). It also blames non-consumers, provided they are still part of the collective who is primarily to blame (ibid.).

Curnutt himself favours a different solution which rests on the claim that drawing personal profit from a morally nefarious practice makes one complicit: "Doing so, and especially doing so when morally innocuous alternatives are readily available, not only indicates support for and the endorsement of moral evil, it is also to participate in that evil. It is an act of complicity" (Curnutt 1997, 166). But this merely shifts the problem by one step: Why does an action 'indicate support for' or 'endorse' moral evil when omitting the action would not have made a difference? Imagine, for example, a meat eater who condemns the evil of the meat industry, campaigns politically against it, and only participates in consuming its products because she firmly believes that individual vegetarianism does not make a difference. Indeed, this activist might argue that vegetarianism is a dangerous pseudo-solution to the evil of the meat industry, because it shifts the view away from system change and towards individual diet change. To claim that this kind of meat eating 'indicates support' for the evils of the meat industry seems plainly ad hoc.[2]

Chignell has proposed a specifically Kantian solution to the causal impotence problem (Chignell 2020), which rests on the view that striving for our own moral perfection requires that we do not let ourselves get demoralised (Chignell 2020, 224). If we take our actions to make no difference in the world, this erodes our resolve to observe our duties (ibid.). So we ought to have faith in the efficacy of our good actions (Chignell 2020, 228). Chignell's solution essentially suggests that even though vegetarians cannot know they are making a difference, they have reason to act *as though* they made a difference, where that reason is based on hope.

However, this argument cannot defuse the causal impotence problem for vegetarians. First, Chignell seems to assume that if *abstaining from meat* makes no difference for animals, then *no action at all* makes a difference. In real life, however, there are many other things people could do to benefit animals, such as supporting animal advocacy and pushing for systemic change. Why, then, should it be so demoralising for vegetarians to accept the inefficacy of vegetarianism, given that there are other ways to make a difference for animals? Secondly, but relatedly, concern for our moral perfection also plausibly requires the opposite of faith in the efficacy of our actions, namely a healthy dose of scepticism and consideration of the available evidence. Demoralisation may be one danger we should avoid for the sake of our moral condition, but wilful ignorance is another. For instance, a good Kantian agent should not wilfully ignore the fact that sending 'thoughts and prayers' to earthquake victims does not make a difference to them. But this seems to be the position in which vegetarians are, according to Chignell's argument. So, while the argument is an intriguing application of a Kantian idea to a real-life conundrum, it is not a satisfactory response to the causal impotence problem.

Even if we ignore the causal impotence problem, other problems plague harm-based arguments. Most importantly, vegetarian arguments focused on the wrongness of inflicting harm might *backfire*. As Bruckner points out, a harm-based argument seems to favour that we eat whatever causes the least harm. Given that harvesting plant-based foods also involves some harm to animals (Bruckner 2016, 35), we avoid the most harm *not* by

---

[2] Another weakness of Curnutt's view is that it cannot easily explain why we should not eat the cow struck by lightning. If there is no wrong involved in the death of an animal, then there is no wrong in which we could make ourselves complicit by profiting from that death.

producing more plant foods, but by deriving as much sustenance as we can from animals who have already died anyway, say, in road accidents (Bruckner 2016, 40). The more of our nutritional need we can meet without killing any more animals, the better.

If Singer, Regan, and Curnutt are right that the principal argument against eating animals revolves around the wrongness of inflicting harm on them, then this argument has no straightforward implications for the morality of ordinary meat eating. We may be obliged to fight for a future in which no more animals are raised and killed for meat, but in the meantime, it makes little difference whether we participate. Harm-based arguments may even demand that we eat some already-dead animals—though not those that are usually eaten—to help spare the lives of others.

One might hope that an argument for vegetarianism has a firmer foothold in Regan's 'respect principle'. The respect principle states that "we are to treat those individuals who have inherent value in ways that respect their inherent value" (Regan 2004, 248). As we have seen in Chap. 8, Regan's idea is that we must not treat beings with inherent value as if they had only instrumental value, neither as a means to our own preconceived ends nor as a means to the maximisation of aggregate pleasure in the world (ibid.). It could be argued that eating someone's dead body just is not respectful in this sense. Some vegetarians certainly think of their refusal to eat animals as a way of honouring or 'respecting' animals' inherent value and of meat eating as an act of instrumentalisation and disrespect.

However, as Fischer has pointed out, "it is a contingent fact about us that we show respect for human beings by not eating their dead bodies" (Fischer 2018, 262). In other words, why does eating someone's dead body necessarily represent a failure to appreciate their inherent value? And why, in the first place, must we express respect for animals by the same behaviour that expresses respect for human beings? At the very least, we must concede that Regan's respect principle is too vague to straightforwardly support a duty of vegetarianism.

The existing literature offers two more, specifically Kantian, arguments against eating animals: One comes from Korsgaard and basically consists in a moral condemnation of what happens in farms and slaughterhouses (Korsgaard 2018, 220–225). What is innovative about her argument is that it sets traditional harm-based arguments on a neo-Kantian foundation. But neither does Korsgaard discuss the causal impotence problem, nor does her approach appear to offer a solution that is not open to other harm-based approaches.

The other Kantian argument for vegetarianism is based on Kant's 'indirect duty' view. Denis puts the point as follows:

Many people become vegetarians as a result of an epiphany in which the fact that animals are killed for (nutritionally unnecessary) meat becomes vivid to them. For them, eating meat would certainly require acting against, and perhaps damaging, their moral sentiments. (Denis 2000, 415)

Denis's central argument is that once we have made the connection between the dead animal on the plate and the once-living animal, our capacity for sympathy is affected. From that point onwards, we have a duty to cultivate our capacity for sympathy by refusing to eat meat.[3] Notice how this argument focuses on the act of meat eating itself. It is not all about the further consequences, about the disutility or the rights violations that may follow from it. Nor is it an argument about complicity through benefitting from a wrong. Denis rather judges the act of meat eating by what it does to the agent. For this reason, Denis's argument is immune to the causal impotence problem, which is a general advantage over harm-based arguments.

However, Denis's 'indirect duty' argument is too fragile to support vegetarianism as a moral cause. It relies on the fact that some people can connect the dead animal to the once-living animal and have a certain affective reaction, but it cannot explain why we *ought* to make this connection or have this reaction. And as Denis herself readily admits, not everybody's sympathy is affected equally (Denis 2000, 415). Most people so far have never had the vegetarian 'epiphany'. What Denis's argument can support, then, is merely a duty of vegetarianism for the particularly perceptive. Counterintuitively, those whose sympathy is already less affected by animals have less of a duty to become vegetarians. The traditional Kantian case for vegetarianism is well-intentioned, but ultimately suffers from the general problem—already discussed in Chap. 3—that it triggers moral duties regarding animals only once we relate to them affectively in a certain way.

The upshot here is emphatically *not* that traditional arguments for vegetarianism are without merit, but that they serve some purposes better

---

[3] Egonsson (1997) put forward essentially the same argument earlier, but in less detail. For this reason, I focus on Denis here. I believe Egonsson's argument has the same strengths and weaknesses as Denis's.

than others. Harm-based arguments are good at stating reasons to move away from harmful animal industries (which was exactly their original purpose in texts like Singer 2002, Regan 2004). But they are not as good at capturing what moves individuals to refuse to eat dead animals. If our goal is to better understand our own ethical outlook, we should be interested in additional argumentative resources.

9.2   A KANTIAN-FOR-ANIMALS ARGUMENT AGAINST EATING ANIMALS

We have seen that traditional arguments for vegetarianism face various difficulties. The most dominant strand of argument, which focuses on the wrongness of inflicting death and suffering on animals, fails because there is only a contingent and complicated relation between harming animals and eating them once they are dead. The Kantian argument offered by Denis fares better in this regard, since it focuses on the act of meat eating itself. This argument however relies entirely on the impact of meat eating on our sympathy, which is also contingent and complicated, and hence cannot robustly ground a duty of vegetarianism.

   I now want to suggest that Kantianism for Animals offers novel resources to address the moral problem of meat eating. In particular, it offers resources to strengthen and clarify a lesser-known consideration against meat eating that is usually couched in more literary language: that a commodifying and mundane treatment of dead bodies violates the "honour of corpses" (Gaita 2002, 44). As Taylor has pointed out, animals are usually considered "ungrievable", and this is one of the ways in which the moral importance of their lives is often downplayed (Taylor 2013, 97). Alas, to my knowledge this line of argument has received no further technical attention in animal ethics. This lack of attention may be due to a central difficulty the argument faces: The dead are beyond harm, so the morality of their treatment appears to be merely a function of our duties to the living (Taylor 2013, 96). But then, to speak of the 'honour of corpses' is merely a roundabout way of speaking about our duties towards living others, and a particularly obscure one at that.

   However, according to Kantianism for Animals, the morality of our treatment of the dead does not have to be a function of our duties towards *other* living beings alone. It may also be a matter of our duties towards self, of our moral perfection. Hence, it makes a crucial difference that

Kantianism for Animals incorporates duties to animals (*pace* traditional Kantianism) as well as duties to self (*pace* dominant approaches to animal ethics). What we need in order to truly capture the 'honour of corpses', I want to suggest, is the notion of *a duty to self which we have only because we also have duties towards others*. We ought to treat the deceased in a certain way, for the sake of our moral condition, *because* they used to be the sort of being towards whom we have duties, until very recently. For convenience's sake, call such duties towards self 'quasi-interpersonal duties', since they are not truly interpersonal (directed towards others), but still hinge on the existence of our duties towards others.

Admittedly, Kant himself does not explicitly introduce or discuss any duties of this kind, even when it comes to the treatment of other human beings. But he clearly sees duties to self and others as intertwined in a way not unlike what I have described. Consider the duty towards self not to lie from the *Doctrine of Virtue*: We have a duty *to self* not to lie, according to Kant's account, because "the dishonour (to be an object of moral contempt) that accompanies it also accompanies a liar, like his shadow" (MM 6:429.11–13). The more general duty at issue here is the duty not to make ourselves the object of contempt in our own eyes, which does not befit the end of our own moral perfection. Evidently, we only make ourselves the object of self-contempt by lying because lying *also* violates a duty towards others. So here we have an example in Kant's framework of a duty towards self which only obtains because we also have a certain duty towards others.

How can the construction of a quasi-interpersonal duty be used to account for the 'honour of corpses'? The straightforward way is to appeal to such duties to justify the claim that we must not *commodify* the dead by treating their bodies *as mundane resources*. That is, because the dead are deceased moral patients towards whom we used to have duties, we ought not to treat the deceased the same way we treat ordinary things. So, while it may *appear* to us as though we had the duty not to eat a dead animal directly towards the animal, we really have this duty towards ourselves. This is an instance of the 'amphiboly in moral concepts of reflection'. At least, that is the broad idea.

Can this line of argument be justified on the basis of Kantianism for Animals? To see to what extent it can, consider Kant's own derivation procedure for duties towards self. As we have seen in Chap. 2, our duties to self stem from the obligatory end of our own moral perfection. For Kant, our moral perfection requires two things: First, as natural beings we ought to keep ourselves in a shape serviceable to morality. Duties of this kind Kant calls 'duties towards self as an animal being'. For instance, we ought not to commit prudential suicide (MM 6:422.03), make ourselves the plaything of our sexual desires (MM 6:424.10), or increase our desires by overindulging in, or even becoming addicted to, food and drugs (MM 6:427.02–03). All of these endeavours would make us worse observers of duties. Secondly, we must act in accordance with the proper self-esteem for our own moral capacities. These Kant calls 'duties towards self purely as a moral being'. The duty not to lie belongs in this category (MM 6:429.02), and Kant adds duties not to be overly frugal (MM 6:432.02) and not to be servile towards others (MM 6:434.20).

So Kant offers two lines of reasoning to justify duties to self: We can show that some endeavour helps in making us good observers of duty, or we can show that it is required as part of the esteem we ought to have for our own moral capacities. Both lines of reasoning can serve as templates for arguments in favour of vegetarianism.

Consider a putative duty to treat recently deceased moral patients in a manner serviceable to our capacity to observe our duties towards the living. Here, we can build on the suggestion that *grief* is the morally appropriate stance towards the recently deceased, including animals (Taylor 2013, 96). Although grief is certainly a complex stance or process, one of its core features is that we regard someone's death as an *important and morally lamentable* event. Death is morally lamentable, but not so much because we can no longer derive pleasure from the company of the deceased. This makes the death of others an *unfortunate* event, but it does not make it morally more significant than other unfortunate events in life.[4] Rather, death is a morally important event because it is the disappearance of a member of the moral community. We can no longer live together in moral relations. In particular, we can no longer partake in moral relations of beneficence (the duty we had towards them, and perhaps they to us), since plainly, there is nothing more we can do to make the deceased happier. Hence, grief is inherently linked to interpersonal moral relations, and grieving is (among other things) a reflection on our moral task. This consideration of death as a morally lamentable event, and the associated

---

[4] I might add that unfortunate events of a certain magnitude can of course be relevant to morality. Some events are so devastating to our happiness that they affect our ability to go about our lives, including the fulfilment of our duties. The death of loved ones can be such an event. However, this does not explain why the death of others is particularly lamentable in case it does not devastate our happiness. It also does not differentiate death from other unfortunate events.

reflection on our duties towards others, is straightforwardly serviceable to morality. We *should* lament it when it becomes impossible to stand in moral relations with others. We should particularly lament it when we can no longer benefit someone. So we plausibly have a duty towards ourselves to grieve for the deceased.

Consider, by contrast, someone who *celebrates* a moral patient's death. It seems straightforward that there is something at least *pro tanto* morally wrong about such a celebration, but there is no harm to the deceased that could account for this wrong. On the account I suggest, celebrating another's death is wrong because in so celebrating, we regard the death of a moral patient—the dissolution of moral relations and the ultimate destruction of their happiness—as a desirable event (although it at least seems to mark it out as important). And treating the bodies of the deceased as a commodity just like any other is only gradually different. From a blasé stance, we regard another's death as morally neutral or unimportant. This is not the stance we ought to take towards death and the dead, *because* we have duties towards the living, particularly the duty to promote their happiness. So we ought not to treat the dead as foodstuffs or other commodities.[5]

The other Kantian argument at our disposal is that treating the dead as foodstuffs does not befit us purely as moral beings. This argument is only plausible if we presuppose that our treatment of the dead is at least a morally delicate affair. Once we presuppose this, however, it seems plausible that esteem for ourselves as moral beings requires that we treat the dead according to *moral* considerations, not *prudential* ones. That is, we ought to exercise control over our conduct in such a morally difficult area. By giving our inclinations free reign over how we treat the dead, we debase ourselves.

It bears emphasising that these duties, like any duty of virtue, do not strictly rule out any specific *act*. They can prohibit certain practical-emotional stances towards the dead and ourselves, from which they and their death appear as banal and unimportant, and from which we appear like inclination-driven automatons unable to exercise moral control over our actions. Neither is compatible with our duties towards self. But there might also be instances of eating corpses where it is not such a casual and

---

[5] As a corollary, this argument implies that we ought not to grieve for things that are *not* moral patients, lest we water down the significance of grief itself. So we ought not to grieve for houseplants and cars, for instance, but we ought to grieve for moral patients.

prudential affair. As Taylor points out, real-life examples come from the world of endocannibalism, the practice of eating the dead of one's own community (Taylor 2013, 89). There have existed societies which treated ingesting the deceased as a ritual of grief. Consider the following account (also referred to by Taylor, ibid.) about the Wari' culture which practised cannibalism until the 1960s:

> Wari' emphasise that they did not eat for self-gratification; indeed, the decayed state of many corpses could make cannibalism quite an unpleasant undertaking. Yet even when the flesh was so putrid that it made them nauseous, some individuals would still force themselves to swallow bits of it. To refuse to consume any of the corpse at all would have been seen as an insult to the dead person's family and to the memory of the deceased. (Conklin 2001, xvii)

Evidently, the Wari' society did not treat the dead casually, nor was their treatment of the dead guided by prudential, inclination-driven considerations. They did not commodify the bodies of the deceased, or otherwise treat them as if they were ordinary things. As Conklin's account makes clear, members of the Wari' society indeed had to *overcome* strong inclinations to observe this grieving practice. By all appearances, eating the recently deceased in this case constitutes *observance* of the duties discussed above, not their violation. Still, if we have these duties, then ordinary meat eating violates them precisely because it is so casual, banal, and inclination-driven. That is not how we ought to treat the bodies of the recently deceased, for our own moral condition's sake. In fact, this is an interesting contrast between the Kantian argument and traditional cases for vegetarianism: Traditional arguments treat the *culinary enjoyment* of meat as a morally innocent pursuit, though it is insufficient to justify the harm to animals on which it depends. According to the Kantian argument, that we eat the dead for the sake of our own culinary enjoyment is constitutive of the wrong at issue.

To summarise, Kantianism for Animals offers an interesting new resource in the debate about vegetarianism, namely the notion of a duty to self which we only have because we also have duties towards others, a quasi-interpersonal duty. Dead animals and human beings are no longer moral patients, but insofar as they *were* moral patients until recently, special duties apply to the treatment of their bodies that are duties towards self. In this way, Kantianism for Animals combines ideas found only separately in the literature up to this point, namely the idea of a duty to self on the one hand, and the idea of a duty towards animals on the other. In this chapter, my aim was to show how Kantianism for Animals brings new resources to the table in debates about vegetarianism. Vegetarian arguments that revolve around the infliction of harm are very limited at best, and counterproductive at worst. While the Kantian proposal is worthwhile that it is duties *to self* that prohibit eating meat, the argument is too weak if it bears no connection at all to duties towards the animals themselves. Kantianism for Animals can appeal to the notion of a quasi-interpersonal duty regarding dead animals: duties we have towards ourselves only because we also have duties towards others. On the conception I have sketched, vegetarianism is obligatory because we have a duty to treat death and the dead as lamentable and important. This is incompatible with a stance that treats the bodies of the deceased as mundane commodities.

Though the argument in this chapter does not condemn all meat eating—again, a certain mode of endocannibalism may be permissible—it does produce a fairly radical argument for vegetarianism. What we usually mean when we talk about 'meat eating' is thoroughly condemned by the argument. And it is an argument which does not hinge on the wrongness of the infliction of death and suffering. Even eating a cow struck by lightning does not appear morally innocuous on the view suggested in this chapter.

References

Bruckner, Donald W. 2016. Strict vegetarianism is immoral. In *The moral complexities of eating meat*, ed. Ben Bramble and Bob Fischer. Oxford: Oxford University Press.

Chignell, Andrew. 2020. Hope and despair at the Kantian chicken factory: Moral arguments about making a difference. In *Kant and animals*, ed. John J. Callanan and Lucy Allais, 213–238. Oxford: Oxford University Press.

Conklin, Beth A. 2001. *Consuming grief: Compassionate cannibalism in an Amazonian society*. Austin: University of Texas Press.

Curnutt, Jordan. 1997. A new argument for vegetarianism. *Journal of Social Philosophy* 28: 153–172.

Denis, Lara. 2000. Kant's conception of duties regarding animals: Reconstruction and reconsideration. *History of Philosophy Quarterly* 17: 405–423.

Diamond, Cora. 1978. Eating meat and eating people. *Philosophy* 53: 465–479.

Egonsson, Dan. 1997. Kant's vegetarianism. *The Journal of Value Inquiry* 31: 473–483.

Fischer, Bob. 2018. Arguments for consuming animal products. In *The Oxford handbook of food ethics*, ed. Anne Barnhill, Mark Budolfson, and Tyler Doggett, 241–263. Oxford: Oxford University Press.

Gaita, Raimond. 2002. *The philosopher's dog.* New York: Routledge.

Hare, Richard M. 1993. Why I am only a demi-vegetarian. In *Essays on bioethics*, 219–236. Oxford: Clarendon Press.

Hudson, Hud. 1993. Collective responsibility and moral vegetarianism. *Journal of Social Philosophy* 24: 89–104.

Korsgaard, Christine M. 2018. *Fellow creatures: Our obligations to the other animals.* Oxford: Oxford University Press.

Regan, Tom. 2004. *The case for animal rights.* Berkeley/Los Angeles: University of California Press.

Singer, Peter. 2002. *Animal liberation.* New York: Ecco Press.

Taylor, Chloe. 2013. Respect for the (animal) dead. In *Animal death*, ed. Jay Johnston and Fiona Probyn-Rapsey, 85–101. Sydney: Sydney University Press.

CHAPTER 10

A Kantian Argument Against Environmental Destruction

10.1   KANT AND THE ENVIRONMENT: PREVIOUS APPROACHES

In Chaps. 8 and 9, I have illustrated how Kantianism for Animals can provide helpful resources to animal ethicists. I have focused on two important issues of animal ethics, the issues of animal use and meat eating. However, the framework's applications are by no means restricted to these topics. In this chapter, I hope to illustrate how Kantianism for Animals can also turn Kant into an interesting, if provocative, interlocutor for environmental ethicists.

In previous debates, Kantians have tried to show that Kant's 'indirect duty' view regarding the environment can produce conclusions similar to those of holistic approaches that assign an inherent moral value to the environment as such, or to ecosystems and species (Altman 2011, 49; see also Lucht 2007; Svoboda 2012, 2014, 2015; Biasetti 2015; Vereb 2019). This is a response to the view Kantians expect environmental ethicists to take, namely that Kant's approach to anything non-human is "ruthlessly exploitative" (Wood 1998, 189). The argument at issue, roughly speaking, is that Kant's approach is not so exploitative after all, particularly if we consider the demands of our duties to self.

Contrary to virtually all contributions on the topic, I hold that this strategy is insufficient to show that traditional Kantianism is not objectionably exploitative towards the environment. Based on cultivation duties

© The Author(s) 2022
N. D. Müller, *Kantianism for Animals*, The Palgrave Macmillan
Animal Ethics Series,
https://doi.org/10.1007/978-3-031-01930-2_10

alone, it is very hard to argue for environmental protections and against the destruction of the environment. The duty Kant and Kantians emphasise most is the duty to cultivate our capacity for aesthetic appreciation. But the existence of this duty does not imply, for instance, that we shouldn't slash-and-burn patches of rainforest to expand industrial feedlots. Only that we should not do it with a lust for wanton destruction. The Kantian contributions to environmental ethics that are enthusiastic about the potential of cultivation duties—while they explore a worthwhile and interesting philosophical move—have generally underestimated the problems posed by Kant's anthropocentrism. Worse yet, by merely reproducing the results of holistic approaches, they obfuscate what could be interestingly different about a Kantian approach that clearly privileges moral patients over the rest of the natural world.

Kantianism for Animals offers an alternative by going the other way: Instead of claiming that its approach to the environment is *not exploitative*, it can argue that once the line of moral concern is moved to include animals, a largely exploitative approach to the unfeeling environment is *not obviously objectionable*. Kantianism for Animals makes it simple to account for rainforest-feedlot cases. But that is simply due to the contingent overlap between our duties to animals and the demands of holistic environmentalism (see Jamieson 1998, 46). We should make no secret of the fact that Kantianism for Animals is a thoroughly individualistic ethical system which demands, for the most part, that we use unfeeling nature as a means to the happiness of animals and human beings. It belongs firmly in the camp of animal liberationist or sentientist ethics, whose contrasts with more holistic environmental ethics are well known (Callicott 1980; Crisp 1998; Varner 2001). But on the one hand, precisely because it is almost unabashedly exploitative of the unfeeling environment, Kantianism for Animals is a more independent, and thus more interesting, Kantian interlocutor position for environmental ethicists. On the other hand, the notion of duties to self helps the framework to avoid some pitfalls of animal liberationist positions in environmental ethics. This makes it all the more helpful to work with.

To start with, consider that environmental ethicists are typically unenthusiastic about Kant. As Rolston puts it, "Kant was still a residual egoist" (Rolston 1988, 340), because he establishes moral principles only between subjects capable of rationally striving for their own happiness and exploiting their environment. Perhaps the most infamous quote of Kant's in environmental ethics is the beginning of the *Anthropology*:

The fact that the human being can have the "I" in his representations raises him infinitely above all other beings on earth. Because of this he is a *person*, and by virtue of the unity of consciousness through all changes that happen to him, one and the same person—i.e., through rank and dignity an entirely different being from *things*, such as irrational animals, with which one can do as one likes. (Anth 7:127.04–10)

In another remark, Kant has an early human being address a sheep with the words: "Nature has given you the skin you wear not for you but for me" (*Muthmaßlicher Anfang* 8:114.07–09). Kant means to say that the human being was right. Now, as we have seen in Chap. 3, his considered view is *not* that human beings can exploit anything non-human in just any way they please. Duties to self demand that we at least conserve our capacity for sympathy and gratitude, hence refrain from acting from cruelty as a motive. Still, it is hard to deny that Kant's remarks express an approach to animals and the environment that is *fundamentally* exploitative. Kant answers the question whether human beings may exploit animals and the environment not with "No", but with "Yes, but...".

In another passage, Kant designates human beings as the 'end of creation':

For what are [animals], together with all the proceeding natural kingdoms, good? For the human being, for the diverse uses which his understanding teaches him to make of all these creatures; and he is the ultimate end of the creation here on earth, because he is the only being on earth who forms a concept of ends for himself and who by means of his reason can make a system of ends out of an aggregate of purposively formed things. (CPJ 5:426.34–427.03)

In this case, however, Kant is not clearly making a moral statement about whether human beings may exploit their environment. The purpose of this passage in the *Critique of the Power of Judgment* is rather to illustrate two kinds of purposiveness (Moyer 2001, 85; see Sect. 6.4). One thing in nature may be 'good for' another like plants are 'good for' herbivores. This is a matter of what Kant calls 'ends of nature' (*Naturzwecke*). Roughly speaking, ends of nature are a matter of ecological and biological functionality (Euler 2015, 2747). In this sense, human beings too are only 'there for' other things in nature, as Kant notes shortly after (CPrR 5:427.11–13; see also MM 6:434.22–25). In the passage quoted, however, Kant means to emphasise that in another sense, everything in nature

224 N. D. MÜLLER

is 'good for', or 'there for' human beings alone. This is so because, to Kant's mind, human beings alone use means to practical ends, while all other animals function purely by instinct and lack instrumental practical reason altogether (see Sect. 6.3). It is only to the human mind that things appear like potential means to ends, Kant holds. So in this sense, all of nature is 'there for' human beings alone, and human beings are right to think of themselves as the end of all creation in this very specific sense.

However, that not all of Kant's statements truly *express* an exploitative attitude towards the non-human environment does not show that Kant's moral philosophy does not *encourage* such an attitude. Setting aside Kant's own stated words, it is easy to construct a Kantian case in favour of an aggressively exploitative stance towards the non-human environment: Kant's moral philosophy demands that we promote the two obligatory ends, which are the happiness of other human beings and our own moral perfection. We ought to use the natural world as a means to these ends. Therefore, while we ought not to exploit nature *selfishly* as a means to our own happiness, we ought to exploit it *to the benefit of other human beings.* This Kantian view prima facie encourages any exploitation of the environment that benefits human beings—even, say, to slash-and-burn a patch of rainforest land to establish a feedlot. And in contrast to a mere *permission* to exploit, this line of reasoning suggests that we have a *duty* to exploit our environment for the benefit of other human beings.

At first glance, then, environmental ethicists would not be wrong to think that Kant's approach to the non-human environment is, at its core, exploitative. Human beings ought to use everything in nature as a means to promote the obligatory ends, and the happiness of other human beings is one of those ends. But if Kant cannot even robustly prohibit slash-and-burn operations in the Amazon rainforest, this presumably amounts to a *reductio* of his view in the eyes of most environmental ethicists.

The objection that Kant licenses and even encourages exploitation of the environment closely resembles the substantive objection to Kant's account of animal ethics (see Sect. 3.3), which claims that Kant licenses indifference to animal suffering. In both cases, Kant is measured against a preconceived moral standard, a standard typically established by appeal to moral intuitions. However, and again in parallel to said debate, the Kantian response to the challenge from environmental ethics has not been to claim immunity against moral intuitions, nor to cast into doubt the specific intuitions with which Kant's view appears to conflict. Rather, Kantians have argued that Kant puts stricter limits on our exploitation of nature than is often acknowledged. Altman even claims that Kant's account, considered in full, has comparable upshots to holistic ethical approaches that assume that the environment has some intrinsic moral value (Altman 2011, 49).

To make this case, traditional Kantians can advance two types of argument: First, they can point out that our duties to other human beings already demand that we do not exploit nature without restriction. Arguing along these lines, Altman emphasises that "[d]irectly harming the environment indirectly harms rational beings" (Altman 2011, 51). Hence, because we have duties to promote the happiness of other human beings, we should not let them be harmed by changes to their environment.

Secondly, Kantians can advance arguments from duties to self regarding our own natural capacities insofar as they are serviceable to morality. Most importantly, Kant encourages us to cultivate our capacity for aesthetic appreciation (MM 6:443.02–09). This is the focus of virtually all Kantian texts on environmental issues (Lucht 2007; Altman 2011; Svoboda 2012, 2014, 2015; Biasetti 2015; Vereb 2019). The capacity for aesthetic appreciation is a capacity to value things disinterestedly (MM 6:443.07–08), which beings like us require to be moral. It is, in effect, a preliminary stage of respect for the moral law, which is also a form of disinterested valuing. So we ought to treat our environment in a way that does not erode our capacity to value things disinterestedly.

However, the import of both types of arguments should not be overstated. Consider first the argument from concern for other human beings. The idea is that what benefits the environment ultimately benefits the human beings in it, and what harms the environment also harms human beings. But this picture itself betrays an anthropocentric bias. As Palmer has pointed out, it is exceedingly hard to tell what might constitute a 'benefit' or 'harm' to such entities as species and ecosystems (Palmer 2011, 277, 280). And whatever we assume to be in the 'interest' of non-human entities, anthropogenic changes to the environment will usually have a diverse range of impacts on them. In other words, the consequences of any change will likely be harmful for some non-human entities in some respects, and beneficial to other entities in other respects. For instance, some ecosystems may wither, collapse, and disappear as a result of anthropogenic climate change, but others will thrive and expand in their place (Palmer 2011, 291). Very often, what we consider to be an 'environmental harm' is simply a change to the environment that may come to harm human beings. In any case, this is the only conception on which the interests of human beings and their environments are *always* aligned.

Of course, the traditional Kantian could move beyond such an anthropocentric conception of environmental harms. But if we define the 'interests' of species and ecosystems without reference to human happiness, there will inevitably arise situations in which things are bad for environments, but good for human beings, and vice versa. Not only does the argument from concern for other human beings suggest that the environment's interests are *overridden* by human interests in such cases, but it implies that the environment's interests do not count for anything at all. So an appeal to duties towards other human beings does not show that Kant's environmental ethic is not exploitative of the non-human environment.

Consider again the rainforest-feedlot example: To slash-and-burn the forest is to destroy part of an ecosystem, which (let us assume) is a 'harm' to it on some non-anthropocentric conception. But to expand the feedlots would promote the happiness of the human beings who stand to gain from it, and its contribution to a longer-term harm to human beings is, at best, uncertain and complicated.[1] So the argument from concern for other human beings finds nothing wrong in expanding the feedlots but may even encourage it.

However, in the debate about Kantian environmental ethics, arguments from concern for other human beings play only a minor role. Much more central are arguments from duties to *self*. Altman claims that the duty to cultivate aesthetic appreciation implies a duty to preserve sublime nature (Altman 2011, 57 f.). This could explain why we should oppose expanding feedlots on rainforest land: The forest is sublime, but the feedlot is not. Therefore, to slash-and-burn the forest to raise the feedlot would be a threat to our capacity for aesthetic appreciation. So we have an indirect duty to refrain from environmental destruction, even though we do not owe this duty to the environment itself.

Three grave problems plague this argument. First, as we have seen, Kant does not just *permit* exploitation of the environment, but plausibly *demands* that we exploit it to the benefit of other human beings. But then, to robustly prohibit slashing-and-burning the rainforest, our duty to cultivate aesthetic appreciation would have to trump our duty of beneficence. There

---

[1] The feedlot may well contribute to anthropogenic climate change which will come to harm human beings. But the feedlot's impact can be set off by other measures, for example by reducing emissions in other sectors of industry. To refrain from constructing the feedlot in the first place is only one, particularly drastic measure.

is no reason to think that it always would. As we saw earlier in Sect. 3.3, the point of cultivating our natural capacities is to enable us to observe our duties. It would be completely wrong headed to prioritise this cultivation over the actual observance of our duties to others. As we also saw, the philosophical primacy that Kant gives to duties to self does not imply a lexical normative primacy. So if Kantians want to argue against the exploitation of the non-human environment, it is not enough for them to merely point out that we have duties to self that conflict with exploitation. They would also have to explain why these specific duties to self should take precedence over our duty to exploit nature to the benefit of other human beings. But there appears to be no reason why they always would.

Secondly, recall from Chap. 3 that Kant's account of animal ethics is good at condemning *intentional* cruelty, but bad at condemning the "legitimate and non-trivial" (Carruthers 2002, 159) motives that drive most violence against animals. A similar problem occurs with regard to the environment: Kant can easily condemn a *"spiritus destructionis"* (MM 6:443.03), a lust for wanton destruction, but he has trouble condemning a somewhat regretful act of destroying sublime nature for the sake of *making a living* or *producing goods for human consumption*. This is more than a mere loophole, given that most environmental destruction today is the result of economic enterprises. It is plainly uncharitable and implausible to suggest that the driver who bulldozes a patch of rainforest is motivated by a lust of wanton destruction, just like most slaughterhouse workers are not motivated by cruelty.

Thirdly, as we have also seen in Chap. 3, things can be good for our capacities that are bad for the objects to which we apply them. In the case of animals, actions that harm animals may help cultivate our sympathy and gratitude, and actions that benefit animals can harm these capacities. The same is true for the environment, assuming that things can 'harm' or 'benefit' it in a non-anthropocentric way.

This point becomes particularly destructive to Kant's view when we consider that nature is not the only source of sublimity in the world. As Kant puts the matter himself, the sublime is "to be sought in our ideas alone" (CPJ 5:250.09). That is, sublimity is not a property of things themselves, but lies in the eye of the beholder. There is no reason, then, why the sublime should be found only in nature. Indeed, some of Kant's own examples of the sublime are artefacts such as the Egyptian pyramids and St Peter's Basilica in Rome (*Beobachtungen* 2:210.09–11). But then, a sublime building may help cultivate our capacity for aesthetic appreciation just as much as the sublime forest which had to be cleared for its construction.

One can press the point even further. Kant points out that the sublime does not have to be pleasant, but it can also be terrifying (*Beobachtungen* 2:209.15). His examples are artistic renderings of a storm and of hell itself (*Beobachtungen* 2:208.27–28). But could there be anything more terrifyingly sublime than the vast, complex, and intricately calculated death machinery of feedlots and slaughterhouses? From a Kantian standpoint, one could argue that appreciating such non-obvious and unsettling sublimity is an even more important moral exercise than appreciating the comparably obvious and pleasant sublimity of rainforests. After all, we thereby cultivate the capacity to value things disinterestedly *at will*, without this valuing having to be triggered by the senses. But then, why oppose the clearing of the rainforest if we can simply appreciate the sublimity of the feedlot more?

The upshot of this section is that it is very difficult for traditional Kantians to argue that Kant's environmental ethic is not objectionably exploitative. Duties to human beings, others or self, only partially mitigate the consequences of Kant's basic commitment to exploitation to the benefit of other human beings. In the next section, I hope to show that Kantianism for Animals provides a worthwhile alternative.

10.2   A KANTIAN-FOR-ANIMALS PERSPECTIVE
ON THE ENVIRONMENT

We have seen that, in response to the objection that Kant's approach to the non-human environment is objectionably exploitative, Kantians have attempted to show that he is not so exploitative after all. However, the arguments they can advance to make this case face serious difficulties. To simply accept Kant's exploitative approach does not seem like an attractive option for Kantians, let alone for most environmental ethicists. However, another option opens up if we accept Kantianism for Animals: Instead of arguing that its approach to the environment is *not exploitative*, we can argue that its exploitation is *not objectionable*. Once we move the line of moral concern to include animals, the demand that we exploit the rest of the natural world for the benefit of moral patients becomes much less repugnant.

More specifically, including animals in moral concern makes a difference to Kantian environmental ethics in three respects: First, it changes what counts as an 'environment'. It is the natural world insofar as it sets conditions for the lives not just of human beings, but of all subjects of happiness. Secondly, it changes what we should consider an 'environmental harm'. What we ought to prevent according to Kantianism for Animals are harms to *subjects of happiness*, not just human beings. Thirdly and perhaps most importantly, including animals in moral concern extends the implications of the Kantian argument that we should protect the environment for the sake of other human beings. Not only must we avoid causing harm to human beings, but also to other animals.

In some cases, the Kantian-for-Animals view produces the conclusions Kantians have previously tried to reach, but for different reasons. For instance, it straightforwardly yields the conclusion that we ought not to slash-and-burn a patch of rainforest in order to build a feedlot. Doing so would violate our duties towards the animals in the forest and those in the prospective feedlot. But of course, this argument does not appeal to any properties of the rainforest that do not affect animals. We ought to exploit the rainforest to the benefit of others, and it just so happens that the best way of doing so is to leave the rainforest as it is—a lot of the time, anyway. So if Kantianism for Animals produces the same results as a holistic approach, it is due to the contingent overlap of the interests of animals and the (arguable) interests of their environments (Jamieson 1998, 46).

For the most part, however, the upshots of Kantianism for Animals are markedly different from those of holistic approaches. It belongs in the camp of animal liberationist or 'sentientist' approaches, and the point is well known in the literature that this camp differs from more holistic approaches (Callicott 1980; Crisp 1998; Varner 2001). Usually, such differences result in objections from the holistic camp to the effect that sentientism cannot account for widely shared environmentalist intuitions. For the rest of this section, let me highlight four major points of disagreement between Kantianism for Animals and holistic approaches, and explain how Kantianism for Animals can avoid some of the associated objections from the holistic camp.

The first and most fundamental difference is that Kantianism for Animals, like any sentientist approach, basically refuses to offer any *independent* considerations in favour of protections for species, ecosystems, biospheres, planets, and so on. Such entities matter morally exactly insofar as they affect the happiness of animals and human beings, plus the moral perfection of human beings.

The traditional main objection against such views is that they prohibit harming individuals for the good of ecosystems, as is the aim in hunting for the sake of population control (Callicott 1980, 312; Varner 2001, 197). Here, Kantianism for Animals largely reproduces the position previously taken by Regan, who denounces hunting as "environmental fascism" (Regan 2004, 362). That is, individuals must not be sacrificed for the sake of ecosystems as such, and this prohibition should not strike us as objectionable. We can try to justify killing individuals by appealing to our duties to others who depend on the stability of the ecosystem, and to an account of why these duties should have priority in a case of apparent moral conflict. But even this could only make killing individuals a means of last resort to be taken with great regret, and the *institution* of hunting as a routine and self-righteous practice is clearly beyond justification for Kantianism for Animals. What the framework can add to Regan's position, however, is that even though we should categorically prioritise individuals over ecosystems, we should still do our best to appreciate the ecosystem's sublimity. We ought to *exploit* the environment, but we ought not to be *callous* towards it. So for instance, we should regret having to let an ecosystem be forever altered or even destroyed by invasive species. So although duties to self do not put any tight restrictions on our treatment of ecosystems, they take the edge off the animal liberationist attitude towards the environment.

Another well-known difference is that holistic approaches to the environment have an easier time justifying duties to *preserve* and *restore* ecosystems, while sentientist approaches must make preservation and restoration contingent on the interests of sentient beings (Varner 2001, 196). Whatever promotes the good of sentient beings, the sentientist approves. Altman intends to side with holists on this matter, deriving a Kantian duty to preserve and restore ecosystems from our duty to appreciate the sublime (Altman 2011, 50). By contrast, Kantianism for Animals sides with sentientism. Whether we ought to preserve, restore, alter, or destroy an ecosystem is largely a matter of our duties towards the animals in and around them. Our duties to self merely put some restrictions on *how* we ought to go about doing whatever is best for the happiness of others. Oftentimes, the best we can do for the animals in an ecosystem is to leave it as it is, and as part of our duties of non-exaltation, we should keep our distance (see Chap. 6). But there is no iron law that non-intervention, or intervention for the sake of preservation and restoration, is always to be favoured. It all depends on the contingent facts of the particular situation. A similar point applies to ongoing environmental *changes*: If Kantianism for Animals demands that we *inhibit or stop* such changes, it is because they are a threat to subjects of happiness. This includes anthropogenic changes just as much as the complex ways in which ecosystems change on their own (see Palmer 2011, 281). But in our assessment whether some given environmental change is a *harm* or *benefit*, we should not be anthropocentric. As Altman correctly points out (Altman 2011, 51 f.), anthropogenic climate change is an anthropocentric environmental harm—a change to the environment of human beings which will harm them. One of the harms he mentions, curiously enough, is that rodents may spread further than before (Altman 2011, 52). This betrays the complications of non-anthropocentric climate ethics: It is not so clear that climate change is more harmful than beneficial to most animals other than human beings (see Palmer 2011, 288). The habitats of some animals will likely shrink and deteriorate, but others will expand and improve. Some animals will lead unhappier and shorter lives, and others happier and longer ones. While Kantianism for Animals by no means licenses a blasé or laissez-faire attitude towards anthropogenic climate change, it calls for a *zoocentric* assessment of its environmental harms and benefits. Zoocentric environmental protection, understood as a moral endeavour to promote and safeguard the happiness of animals and human beings, should begin with the dismantling of systems of animal exploitation, which after all inflict deliberate and immediate harm on animals.

What Kantianism for Animals can add to the sentientist position is, once again, the contention that our duties to self nevertheless demand that we cultivate appreciation for the sublime in nature. Though this does not require that we preserve and restore ecosystems across the board, it demands that we do not indulge in a *spiritus destructionis* when we alter the environment for the sake of moral patients.

A third difference between holism and sentientism is that holists can easily account for the intuition that the last person on earth should not wantonly destroy an ecosystem, assuming there are no sentient beings left in it (Varner 2001, 200). To a sentientist, who holds that literally *all* our duties hinge on the interests of sentient beings, it would seem that this destruction is permissible. Evidently, Kantianism for Animals is

232 N. D. MÜLLER

well-equipped to deal with this case. *Wanton* destruction is opposed to a duty we have towards *self*, and the last person on earth would have it against themselves too. However, once again we need not exaggerate the import of this duty. If the last person on earth had any non-trivial reason for destroying the ecosystem, and destroyed it with appropriate regret, Kantianism for Animals would not forbid it. But this position does not seem objectionable.

Last but not least, an important difference between Kantianism for Animals and holism is that according to Kantianism for Animals, no moral merit attaches to environmental action that is isolated from practical benevolence. Its main line of reasoning in favour of environmental protection is that we *ought* to exploit the unfeeling environment to the benefit of moral patients, *but* that overexploitation may backfire and harm the moral patients we ought to benefit. But then, our environmental efforts can *only* be moral if they occur against the backdrop of a project that aims at the happiness of human beings and animals. Environmental action for the sake of species and ecosystems *alone* is not what duty demands. From the perspective of Kantianism for Animals, such environmental action is philosophically confused. Worse yet, it is likely to be driven purely by inclination—perhaps an inclination to enjoy the beautiful and sublime in nature, or an inclination to secure the future of one's own offspring. To act on these inclinations while ignoring our duties towards animals is straightforwardly immoral. So Kantianism for Animals emphatically calls for a *zoocentric environmentalism*, dismissing or even condemning any form of anthropocentric or holistic environmentalism that does not oppose the exploitation of animals.

To sum up, in this chapter, I have argued that traditional Kantianism is fundamentally exploitative of the non-human environment. Though Kantians are right to point out that harms to environments oftentimes also harm human beings, and that we have duties to self to cultivate our capacity to appreciate the sublime, these arguments do not plausibly condemn most actual environmental destruction for human gain.

The key to a more robust Kantian condemnation of environmental destruction is to move the line of moral concern to include animals. Although Kantianism for Animals is still fundamentally exploitative, it is only exploitative of the *unfeeling* environment to the benefit of *beings capable of happiness*, who are animals and human beings. Environmental protections, but also active changes to the environment, are called for exactly to the extent that they prevent an overexploitation that backfires, harming subjects of happiness. However, Kantianism for Animals does not offer any considerations that favour environmental protections independently of their impact on animals and human beings. This leads to a thoroughly zoocentric environmentalism that puts different demands on us than either an anthropocentric approach or a non-anthropocentric approach that assigns value to species, ecosystems, and other unfeeling entities. In particular, Kantianism for Animals requires that environmental efforts must be connected to practical benevolence towards others, so that concern for the environment *as detached from* concern for animals appears non-moral or even immoral.

REFERENCES

Altman, Matthew C. 2011. *Kant and applied ethics: The uses and limits of Kant's practical philosophy*. Malden, MA: Wiley-Blackwell.

Biasetti, Pierfrancesco. 2015. From beauty to love: A Kantian way to environmental moral theory? *Environmental Philosophy* 12: 139–160.

Callicott, J. Baird. 1980. Animal liberation: A triangular affair. *Environmental Ethics* 2: 311–338.

Carruthers, Peter. 2002. *The animals issue: Moral theory in practice*. Cambridge: Cambridge University Press.

Crisp, Roger. 1998. Animal liberation is not an environmental ethic: A response to Dale Jamieson. *Environmental Values* 7: 476–478.

Euler, W. 2015. Zweck. In M. Willaschek, J. Stolzenberg, G. Mohr, & S. Bacin (Eds.), *Kant-Lexikon* (pp. 2745–2753). De Gruyter.

Jamieson, Dale. 1998. Animal liberation is an environmental ethic. *Environmental Values* 7: 41–57.

Lucht, Marc. 2007. Does Kant have anything to teach us about environmental ethics? *American Journal of Economics and Sociology* 66: 127–149.

Moyer, Jeanna. 2001. Why Kant and ecofeminism don't mix. *Hypatia* 16(3): 79–97.

Palmer, Clare. 2011. Does nature matter? The place of the nonhuman in the ethics of climate change. In *The ethics of global climate change*, ed. Denis G. Arnold, 272–291. Cambridge: Cambridge University Press.

Regan, Tom. 2004. *The case for animal rights*. Berkeley/Los Angeles: University of California Press.

Rolston, Holmes. 1988. *Environmental ethics: Duties to and values in the natural world*. Philadelphia: Temple University Press.

Svoboda, Toby. 2012. Duties regarding nature: A Kantian approach to environmental ethics. *Kant Yearbook* 4: 143–163.

Svoboda, Toby. 2014. A reconsideration of indirect duties regarding non-human organisms. *Ethical Theory and Moral Practice* 17: 311–323.

Svoboda, Toby. 2015. *Duties regarding nature*. New York: Routledge.

Varner, Gary. 2001. Sentientism. In *A companion to environmental philosophy*, ed. Dale Jamieson, 192–203. Malden, MA: Wiley-Blackwell.

Vereb, Zachary T. 2019. *The case for the green Kant: Defense and application of a Kantian approach to environmental ethics*. Doctoral dissertation, University of South Florida.

Wood, Allen W. 1998. Kant on duties regarding non-rational nature. *Aristotelian Society Supplementary Volume* 72: 189–210.

CHAPTER 11

Animal Ethics and the Philosophical Canon: A Proposal

In this book I have proposed a Kantian view which includes animals in moral concern, not by adding a new line of reasoning to the existing Kantian corpus, but by making changes to Kant's conception of moral concern. The resulting system, called Kantianism for Animals, retains core features of Kant's views in moral philosophy: As rational beings, we autonomously impose the moral law on ourselves. This law marks out two ends as obligatory, namely others' happiness and our own moral perfection. From these obligatory ends, we can derive materially specific duties. In these respects, nothing at all has been changed about Kant's philosophy. However, Kantianism for Animals is a somewhat unorthodox version of Kantianism in three respects:

First, it views the Formula of Humanity, along with other formulations of the Categorical Imperative, *not* as a substantive moral principle, but purely as a formal principle of autonomous willing. It is not a principle to which we should turn in order to arrive at specific ethical action-guidance. Frankly, the Categorical Imperative plays only a minor role if our interest lies in determining *what* a good will wills, not *how* it wills. To arrive at specific action-guidance, we should move from the idea of a good will to the doctrine of obligatory ends, and from there to specific ethical duties. The crucial question when it comes to animals is therefore not 'Are they ends in themselves?', but rather, 'Should their happiness be promoted as part of the obligatory ends?' As I hope to have shown, it is much easier to argue for an affirmative answer to the latter question than to the former.

© The Author(s) 2022   235
N. D. Müller, *Kantianism for Animals*, The Palgrave Macmillan
Animal Ethics Series,
https://doi.org/10.1007/978-3-031-01930-2_11

Secondly, any 'second-personal' element has been removed from Kant's system. The existence of duties towards others does *not* depend on the capacity to 'constrain' each other under a mutually shared moral law. Kantianism for Animals locates the normative basis of our duties in the autonomy of the moral agent alone, with none of the normative work being left to any supposed authority of others. Duties are directed 'towards' others, on the alternative view I have put forward, simply in the sense that they are duties derived from the obligatory end of the happiness of others. So the directionality of our duties hinges on *what* they ask us to do and *why*. Admittedly, this conception does not produce *exactly* the same upshots as more second-personal approaches when it comes to moral practices like consenting, apologising, and forgiving. But the differences are smaller than one might expect, and they are not obviously objectionable.

Third, some changes were made to Kant's conception of duties to others. The type of duty to others which could only plausibly hold vis à vis human beings—duties of respect—was recategorised as a duty to self, merely *regarding* others. It is basically a duty not to exalt ourselves above others, and this duty we must observe even in our beneficence towards others. Finally, an expansion was made to Kant's conception of animal agency. Although animals do not pursue their happiness as a matter of instrumental reason, they have a greater extent of goal-orientation than Kant acknowledged. The goals they pursue also *indicate* their happiness, even if they are not purposefully chosen as means to happiness. Hence, duties of love towards animals, like Kant's duties of love to human beings, demand primarily that we help along another's self-chosen endeavours. This retains the anti-paternalistic flavour of Kant's account of beneficence.

One aim of this book was to show that the deviations it takes to make Kantianism include animals in moral concern are more peripheral than one might think. We need not abandon the core of Kant's system, such as the view that morality arises from autonomy, not pleasure and pain, or compassion. The most substantial point of disagreement with Kant is on an issue he himself only considers in passing, namely his account of interpersonal ethical obligation. As long as we insist that such obligation exists only given mutual 'necessitation' or 'constraint' under a shared moral law, animals will inevitably be excluded from the moral universe. But nothing more central in Kant's ethical system forces us to adopt this view. With the purely first-personal view, an alternative is open to us. So Kant is much closer to including animals in moral concern than animal ethicists often suppose.

The other aim was to provide a novel system to animal ethicists that helps them reflect on our moral relations to animals. Kant's moral philosophy amounts to more than a *claim*. It comprises its own set of questions, answers, notions, distinctions, and arguments. It lays different emphases and tells different stories than other approaches. My hope is that having this approach in the philosophical toolbox will help to advance the thought of animal-friendly ethicists and philosophically interested animal advocates.

At the outset of this book, I have characterised its approach as *constructive* and *revisionist*, and I have presupposed a *radical* agenda. It is an approach that treats Kant not as a philosophical authority, but as a philosophical resource. Hopefully, the project can serve as a proof of concept for this kind of approach to the canon. In principle, one can apply it to any and all philosophers, particularly to those whose thought is usually understood to be highly systematic, but inimical to the moral claims of animals. Why not take the same approach to Spinoza, for example?[1] Or Habermas?[2] Or Rawls?[3] Having applied the approach to Kant, let me highlight some reasons why this research programme could be worthwhile.

First, recall that one motivating reason for this project was that Kant's moral philosophy should not be left to those who want to diminish or dismiss the moral claims of animals (see Chap. 1). I hope to have shown that Kant's exclusion of animals does not stem from what is usually considered to be the core of his system. In particular, the view that morality arises from autonomy does not commit us to Kant's claim that there can be duties only towards autonomous beings. If we prefer, we can even double down on Kant's view that the moral law is autonomously self-imposed to remove all second-personal elements from his ethical theory. So it is not *in spite of* Kant's view that morality arises from autonomy that we can account for duties towards non-moral beings, but *because* of it. This shows how a

---

[1] For a critical contribution on Spinoza's animal ethics see Grey (2013). However, a constructive, revisionist, radical approach could hopefully reveal more of a positive potential of Spinoza's thought for progressive animal ethicists.

[2] Whitworth (Whitworth 2002) briefly explores the possibility of including nature in Habermas's thought. It would be worthwhile, however, to see whether a Habermasian can draw any meaningful ethical distinction between animals and the rest of nature.

[3] Abbey (Abbey 2007) considers the resources Rawls provides to animal ethics as-is. Rowlands (Rowlands 1998) takes a more revisionist approach in reconsidering *pace* Rawls which features ought to be unknown behind the veil of ignorance (Rowlands 1998, 142–152). This may be the clearest example of a constructive, revisionist, radical approach to a philosophical classic, but Rowlands's relatively brief treatment of the topic still leaves much to explore.

constructive, revisionist, radical approach can help us lay claim to ideas that are usually left to those opposed to stronger concern for animals.

Secondly, the project has shown that a constructive, revisionist, radical approach can also be interesting from an exegetical perspective. Not only does such an approach lead us to emphasise different questions than other contributions to the literature, but it often leads us to consider familiar questions from a different angle and make new connections. Case in point: The literature discusses the question to what extent the Formula of Humanity should be understood as a substantive moral principle (Reath 2013; see Chap. 4). But it was only during the search for Kantianism for Animals that this question turned out to have crucial implications for who matters morally. The further we remove the Categorical Imperative from direct action-guidance, the greater the prospect of including those who do not share the moral law. This also shows how exegetical issues are not always as morally innocent as they seem at first sight.

In other cases, what is primarily discussed as a problem or difficulty has turned out to be a positive resource for theory-modification. For instance, the literature discusses Thompson's puzzle mostly as a difficulty for Kantian moral philosophers (Thompson 2004; Fanselow 2008; Darwall 2009; Palatnik 2018; see Chap. 5). In this debate, Kantians have something to lose—the plausibility of their ethical framework—and little to win. But in the present project, the puzzle has inspired the purely first-personal 'content approach' to moral directionality. So taking a constructive, revisionist, and radical approach can make visible a surprising creative potential.

Third, I hope that the book's last part has illustrated what animal ethics has to gain from the modification and repurposing of ethical systems. By asking what it would take to include animals in moral consideration in a system that originally excluded them, we can gain new and unfamiliar perspectives on our moral relations to animals. I have highlighted that Kantianism for Animals can be used to criticise the practical-emotional stances towards animals inherent in our conduct. The framework condemns the stance from which we treat our own ends as overriding our duty to promote the happiness of animals, which leads to a novel, motive-oriented argument against animal use. It also offers novel possibilities because it combines concern for the happiness of others with concern for our own moral perfection, which can help account for the problematic nature of practices which do not directly harm animals. According to the argument I have proposed, eating meat violates a duty to self which we have only because we have duties towards animals. I have also highlighted that the framework has quite distinct upshots for environmental ethicists than other approaches. It enables a zoocentric critique of both anthropocentric and holistic environmentalism that can, at the very least, be an independent and interesting interlocutor position in environmental ethics.

Most fundamentally, however, repurposing Kant for animal ethics has produced a framework with an unfamiliar *mission statement*. Kantianism for Animals does not primarily aim at investigating what we ought to do, particularly in situations of moral conflict (an issue on which it is, like Kant, admittedly unclear). Kantianism for Animals instead aims to address the predicament of the ordinary moral agent—of feeling the pressure of duty yet being tempted to pursue inclination instead. It responds to this predicament with a positive account of what our duties demand and how they can demand it. It vindicates the duties we already take ourselves to be having most of the time and helps to safeguard us against the corrosive influence of self-serving rationalisations. This shows how reconsidering past philosophers can even reveal new practical purposes for animal ethics itself.

Turning back to Kantian animal ethics, the present project must leave some questions open. For one thing, the Kantian-for-Animals framework inherits some vaguenesses from Kant. Again, it does not give clear guidance on how to deal with moral conflicts, since Kant himself says lamentably little about this topic (Timmermann 2013, 36). So while Kantianism for Animals demands that we promote the happiness of others, it does not spell out what this means in cases where the happiness of one conflicts with the happiness of others. In such cases, there are two things we can do: First, we can take Kant's silence as a reminder that moral philosophy *can* do other things besides resolving conflicts between putative duties (see Sect. 2.6); secondly, we can extend and modify the framework further. For instance, one could develop an account of moral conflict-resolution starting from Kant's claim that *duties* cannot conflict, only their *grounds* (MM 6:224.17–21). While this book could only establish the bare bones of Kantianism for Animals, the framework is open to further specifications and modifications.

Admittedly, the project also makes a major omission that it does not inherit from Kant, since it does not cover duties of right (see Sect. 1.3). More work is needed to investigate what options are open to Kantian ethicists to account for legal protections for animals. If we take Kant's philosophy as-is, it would appear that such protections are undermotivated, especially if they restrict the external freedom of human beings. But surely, the implication must strike many readers as morally repugnant, or indeed as absurd, that legal animal protections ought to be abolished out of respect for a putative freedom to abuse. What is more, the considerations in Chaps. 3 and 10 should caution us against exaggerated enthusiasm for 'indirect duty' views. Each time they have been offered, these positions turned out to be full of loopholes and exhibit considerable weaknesses. To secure a robust basis for legal animal protections in Kantianism, we must find some way to establish duties of right towards animals. Hence, there should be an interest on the part of both animal ethicists and Kantian ethicists to devote more attention to this topic.

Another limitation is that the present project *proposed* a system without doing much to *defend* it. On the one hand, there may be objections from moral intuition, according to which Kantianism for Animals has unacceptable implications. Seeking a reflective equilibrium between the Kantian framework and moral intuitions was never Kant's goal, nor was it mine in this book. But to object to some of the framework's upshots and then modify its claims to find an equilibrium can still be fruitful for theory-formation in animal ethics. Kantianism for Animals is not intended to be the final destination of moral theory. It is another 'base camp' from which to launch theoretical expeditions.

On the other hand, there may be theoretical objections from the perspective of other approaches. Though I have pointed out differences between Kantianism for Animals and utilitarianism and various views in animal and environmental ethics (Chaps. 7, 8, 9, and 10), I have not always provided an explanation why it is Kantianism for Animals that should strike us as more compelling. This kind of juxtaposition and comparative evaluation can be just as worthwhile as testing Kantianism for Animals against moral intuitions. The point of this book was to put Kantianism for Animals on the table in the first place.

Finally, it has become clear over the course of this book that there are many more issues on which a Kantian-for-Animals position can be developed. By discussing animal use, meat eating, and environmental protections, I have picked out three issues that are particularly prominent and important. But of course, I have left out many others. What might a Kantian-for-Animals say about animal euthanasia, wild animal suffering, moral education regarding animals, the ethics of captivity, or pet-keeping? I hope to have shown that Kantianism for Animals offers abundant resources to tackle such issues and that the views it produces are often original, stringent, and compelling.

REFERENCES

Abbey, Ruth. 2007. Rawlsian resources for animal ethics. *Ethics and the Environment* 12: 1–22.

Darwall, Stephen. 2009. Why Kant needs the second-person standpoint. In *The Blackwell guide to Kant's ethics*, ed. Thomas E. Hill, 138–158. Malden, MA: Wiley-Blackwell.

Fanselow, Ryan. 2008. A Kantian solution to Thompson's puzzle about justice. *Proceedings of the XXII World Congress of Philosophy* 10: 91–99.

Grey, John. 2013. "Use them at our pleasure": Spinoza on animal ethics. *History of Philosophy Quarterly* 30: 367–388.

Palatnik, Nataliya. 2018. Kantian agents and their significant others. *Kantian Review* 23: 285–306.

Reath, Andrews. 2013. Formal approaches to Kant's formula of humanity. In *Kant on practical justification*, ed. Mark Timmons and Sorin Baiasu, 201–228. Oxford: Oxford University Press.

Rowlands, Mark. 1998. *Animal rights: Moral theory and practice*. New York: Palgrave Macmillan.

Thompson, Michael. 2004. What is it to wrong someone? A puzzle about justice. In *Reason and value: Themes from the moral philosophy of Joseph Raz*, ed. R. Jay Wallace, Philip Pettit, Samuel Scheffler, and Michael Smith, 333–384. Oxford: Oxford University Press.

Timmermann, Jens. 2013. Kantian dilemmas? Moral conflict in Kant's ethical theory. *Archiv für Geschichte der Philosophie* 95: 2013.

Whitworth, Andrew. 2002. Communication with the environment? Non-human nature in the theories of Jürgen Habermas. *Politics* 20: 145–151.

Index[1]

[1] Note: Page numbers followed by 'n' refer to notes.

Printed by Printforce, the Netherlands